# The Vital Psoas Muscle

## Connecting Physical, Emotional, and Spiritual Well-Being

**Jo Ann Staugaard-Jones**

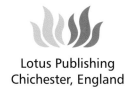

Lotus Publishing
Chichester, England

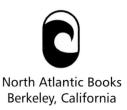

North Atlantic Books
Berkeley, California

First published in 2012 by
**Lotus Publishing**
Apple Tree Cottage, Inlands Road, Nutbourne, Chichester, PO18 8RJ and
**North Atlantic Books**
P. O. Box 12327
Berkeley, California 94712

**Drawings** Amanda Williams, Pascale Pollier
**Text Design** Wendy Craig
**Cover Design** Paula Morrison
**Printed and Bound** in the UK by Scotprint

*The Vital Psoas Muscle: Connecting Physical, Emotional, and Spiritual Well-Being* is sponsored by the Society for the Study of Native Arts and Sciences, a nonprofit educational corporation whose goals are to develop an educational and cross-cultural perspective linking various scientific, social, and artistic fields; to nurture a holistic view of arts, sciences, humanities, and healing; and to publish and distribute literature on the relationship of mind, body, and nature.

**British Library Cataloguing-in-Publication Data**
A CIP record for this book is available from the British Library
ISBN 978 1 905367 24 5 (Lotus Publishing)
ISBN 978 1 58394 458 5 (North Atlantic Books)

**Library of Congress Cataloguing-in-Publication Data**
Staugaard-Jones, Jo Ann.
  The vital psoas muscle: connecting physical, emotional, and
spiritual well-being / Jo Ann Staugaard-Jones.
      p. ; cm.
  Includes bibliographical references.
  Summary: "Full-color alternative approach to understanding and
balancing the most important skeletal muscle in the body, aimed at the
layperson as well as the professional body practitioner concerned with
core strengthening and psoas-related back, hip, knee, and pelvic tension
issues"--Provided by publisher.
  ISBN 978-1-58394-458-5
  I. Title.
  [DNLM: 1. Lumbosacral Region--physiology. 2. Psoas Muscles--physiology.
3. Exercise Movement Techniques. 4. Mind-Body
Therapies. 5. Muscle Stretching Exercises. WE 750]

  613.7'18--dc23
                        2011036026

# Contents

# Foreword

I have had the pleasure of knowing and working with Jo Ann for approximately ten years and have the utmost respect for someone who epitomizes health and fitness in thought, word, and deed. She has touched many lives as a teacher and professor, and again as an author in writing her second book. When she asked me to contribute to this book, I was both humbled and honored. When she told me the topic of the book, I was excited. Having spent over 24 years in clinical practice, I have my share of "psoas stories" and I clearly knew the importance of this often-overlooked muscle. However, after reading the book, I was again humbled at my limited knowledge of how all-encompassing this muscle is. Being in active clinical practice, I love courses and books that have a profound impact on my thinking and that influence the way I treat my patients Monday morning. *The Vital Psoas Muscle* is most definitely one of those books.

The psoas muscle can be considered a realtor's dream, in that it's all about *location, location, location*! Due to its location, the psoas has the unique distinction of being the only muscle that connects the upper body to the lower body. Therefore the functional ramifications are vast, with the muscle acting as either a prime mover of the action or a critical stabilizer in concert with other prime movers. So whether the movement is lower-quarter driven in a function such as walking, or more upper-quarter driven in a movement such as throwing a ball or reaching upward to an overhead cabinet, the psoas is working. Many clinicians respect the ability of the psoas to function as a prime mover involved in hip flexion; however, despite knowing its proximal attachments to the anterior aspects of the lumbar spine and numerous fascial relationships, they often overlook its function as a *stabilizer*, as well as its ability to profoundly affect posture.

The location of the psoas also affords it the ability to influence *circulation*, due to its anatomic proximity to vascular structures, particularly the aorta and the external iliac artery and its continuation into the femoral artery through the complex ilioinguinal area. The psoas possesses crucial fascia connections to support numerous visceral structures and organs. These same organs, through muscular contraction of the psoas, can be stimulated and "massaged" and subsequently exert influences on the digestion, excretion/elimination, detoxification, and even reproduction processes of the body. The psoas affects *respiration* via its anatomic relationship with the diaphragm in the area of the solar plexus, which also then influences *energy flow* throughout the body through its geographic relationship to the lower three chakras of yoga philosophy. Jo Ann does a beautiful job of touching upon the psoas's influence on such topics as "visceral messaging" and "somatic memory," as well as the *emotional* component associated with our "gut feelings."

Jo Ann addresses the meaning of "wheel" for the word *chakra*. It would not be inconceivable to place the psoas as the hub of that wheel, with a few of the many spokes that are driven and influenced by that hub being our upper body, lower body, core, physiologic and metabolic functions, emotions, spirit, and energy, to name just a few. She has also educated us that the historical meaning of chakra is "to bring about a new age." After digesting and assimilating the factual information, as well as offering a functional demonstration of the corrective, rebalancing exercises and practices, our author has provided us with a valuable roadmap for the restoration of harmony between the mind, body, and spirit through this deeply hidden treasure known as the psoas. I think clinicians, anatomists, bio-mechanists, exercise specialists, massage therapists, and others will most certainly be brought to a "new age" of awareness, recognition, acceptance, and respect for this deeply centered muscle's ability to concomitantly affect the mind, the body, and the spirit. It is a widely held belief that only through the balance of all three can optimal health be achieved.

My final reflection is on Jo Ann's indication that "as the universe is interrelated, so is our body; we are life forms constantly evolving." This book has enlightened and assisted me in my own personal and professional evolutionary process, and I feel that any reader, after taking this journey with the author, will be able to add a layer of knowledge and enlightenment on their own path to a better understanding of optimal health and function.

In health,
**Dr. Gary Mascilak**, D.C., P.T., C.S.C.S

# Introduction

*The Vital Psoas Muscle* was written because it explains the only muscle in the human organism that connects the upper body to the lower body. Most people are not actually aware of how important this is.

In teaching and researching the psoas as a major force in the body, I began a journey from the kinesiological point of view, into the realm of body flow, energies, and proprioception. This experience has humbled me.

**Physically**: As a movement specialist I found the mechanics documented, as recently as a year ago, in a state of flux as to psoas actions and roles. Renowned psoas experts are constantly updating information to help sort everything out. The most simplified statement is this: *the psoas is complicated*. No longer will I call the psoas a major mover of hip flexion, except as part of the iliopsoas muscle group, where the iliacus is the stronger flexor in most cases. In the lumbar spine, there are other muscles that remain the more powerful flexors, mainly the rectus abdominis. The roles of the psoas major as both a lumbar spine and hip stabilizer and a connector to the lower extremity appear more important mechanically and warrant its significance, yet its stabilizing functions are still in question depending on the movement.

**Emotionally**: In the field of psycho-emotional connection, information on the psoas's relation with the nervous system is mind-boggling, yet very real. I have tried to make this material accessible to a larger audience in a way it can be understood.

**Spiritually**: Knowledge of spiritual energies has been mostly examined through ancient texts and the science of Kundalini yoga and meditation, which appear thorough and relevant to this day. The psoas remains an important figure within this realm because of its deep location, central placement, and relation to other structures. Even though the "subtle" body is thought of as separate from the anatomical structure, the two are truly related, for how can energy flow without breath and muscular work serving in some way? The skill is in the perception. As the universe is interrelated, so is the body; we are life forms constantly evolving.

How we use the psoas and take care of it is crucial. Everyone is different, but its misuse is overwhelmingly apparent in many people. The psoas has become an innocent culprit in various situations, some explained in this text. Finding a specialist who can diagnose and deal with the psoas is difficult. Treatment and commitment to healing can be frustrating, yet effective, as the psoas is restored to its full potential.

I have found that *freeing* the psoas is more directly a complement to the full body system, with strengthening or stretching secondary, in many cases. This is because the psoas is not just misused – it is abused. Once released it can operate effectively in the very important roles discussed in this book. I love the words used by Liz Koch, an extraordinary psoas expert: "juicy, responsive, supple." If followed, these words can lead to a healthy psoas that affects so many important modalities in the body.

**Jo Ann Staugaard-Jones**
movetolive.joannjones@gmail.com

# Part 1:
# Anatomical Prelude

This text is an attempt to decipher one important muscle, when it is clear that no one muscle works alone. The core area is made up of a group of muscles that girdle the spine to hold it in balance. The psoas major is one of these muscles, and is aided by the rectus abdominis, obliques, transversus abdominis, latissimus dorsi, erector spinae, quadratus lumborum, and deep posterior muscles to stabilize the lower spine. At the iliofemoral joint, it is part of the iliopsoas muscle group, which works with the rectus femoris, sartorius, pectineus, and tensor fasciae latae to flex the hip. With all these muscles helping, the psoas major can be free to perform a most significant function: integral connection.

In this age of core fitness, it is important to remember that all central muscles must be in harmony with each other, and that no one muscle is emphasized. Many fitness instructors rely on the "naval to spine" phrase, mostly to engage the deep transversus abdominis. One must realize that this is only an image, and must not be used in excess to hollow the abdominals or press the back flat. The best alignment in movement is the neutral spine, where the natural spinal curves balance each other and allow the muscles to lithely do their jobs.

With this in mind, the anatomical part of the book can begin.

# 1

# Anatomy and Biomechanics of the Psoas Area

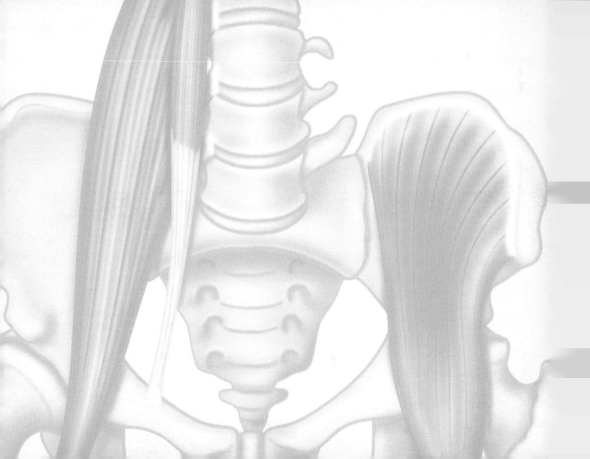

## The Iliopsoas Muscle Group: Location and Actions

Deep within the anterior hip joint and lower spine lies the **psoas major** muscle. Sometimes called the "mighty psoas," *it is the most important skeletal muscle in the human body*, as it is the only muscle that connects the upper extremity to the lower extremity (the spine to the legs). This makes it a very significant postural muscle and mover and stabilizer of two different joints: the iliofemoral joint and the lumbar spine. The muscle is also located near the body's center of gravity, so its role becomes that of regulating balance, and affecting nerve and subtle energies as well.

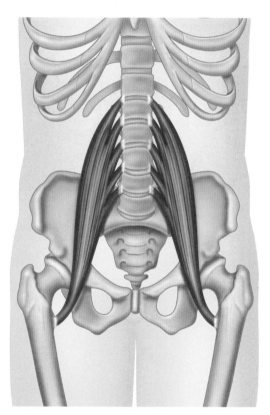

*Figure 1.1: Psoas major.*

The **psoas** has a **major** and a **minor** muscle, mostly synergistic at the lumbar spine. The difference is in their distal attachments: the major is the one that connects the femur to the spine (lower to upper extremities); the minor connects the pelvis to the spine. Some say the minor will become extinct, as it was important when humans walked on four legs, and not necessarily needed now. It is also a very weak mover. In fact, some people only have it on one side, or do not have it at all. When only the word "psoas" is used, it is generally understood to be the psoas major, or a combination of the major and minor as one muscle group.

Do not pronounce the "p" – phonetically it is "so-az."

Both psoas muscles are part of a larger muscle group called the **iliopsoas**, which also includes the large **iliacus**. This group, contracting simultaneously, flexes the hip. It is the deepest of the hip flexors, and possibly the strongest as a muscle group. The iliacus attaches from the femur to the iliac bone of the pelvis, while the psoas major distally attaches to the femur, and proximally (nearest to the center of the body) attaches past the pelvis to the transverse processes of the first through fifth lumbar vertebra and sometimes the twelfth thoracic vertebra. Most sources have stated this allows at least part of the psoas to flex the lumbar spine, although it is being debated. If the femur is fixed, the iliacus will act at the pelvis, while the psoas may work on the lumbar spine. It can even use its lumbar fibers to extend the spine. This contradiction is explained in more detail later.

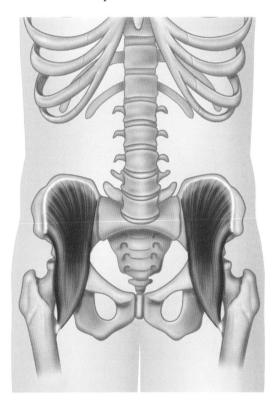

*Figure 1.2: Iliacus.*

The iliacus can also aid the pelvis in tilting forward, along with other hip flexors such as the rectus femoris. This forward tilt has a tendency to enhance lumbar *lordosis* (anterior curving of the spine), so the psoas must be strong yet pliant enough to help stabilize the area from too much advanced lordosis, or "sway back," one of the most common conditions of poor posture. The abdominals can also help counteract this (specifically the rectus abdominis), as can the spinal extensors. The psoas becomes its own antagonist in stabilization between lumbar spine flexion and extension.

> *Centering the pelvis with muscles other than the psoas major and maintaining neutral (natural) spinal curves is key to allowing the psoas to do its many jobs without fatigue.*

Research suggests that the psoas muscles, by forming a muscle bundle around the lumbar spine with the lower **transversospinalis** muscles (see figure 1.5), can help erect the lower spine, while other fibers can flex the area. Either way, as a core muscle the psoas is a force in correct body alignment. It is also of utmost importance in the transfer of weight through the trunk to the legs and feet while moving (and even when standing), as it helps to position the spine, pelvis, and femur in relation to one another.

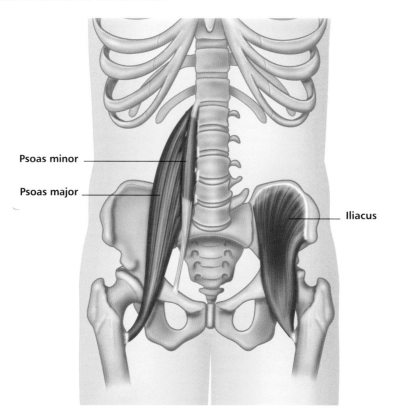

Psoas minor

Psoas major

Iliacus

*Figure 1.3: The iliopsoas muscle group. Imagine the muscle structure on both sides of the body to realize the full extent of the group.*

The deep yet powerful three-muscle group of the iliopsoas working together can bring the thigh anteriorly (flexion of the hip), along with other anterior hip muscles. When the pelvis is stationary, one can isolate the psoas major by lifting the leg up in front of the body, as in the sitting "V-position." With gravity as resistance, this engages the psoas in strong support of the lumbar spine, as well as some minor work at the hip.

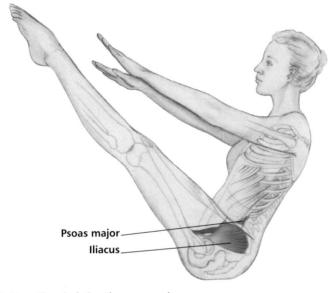

Psoas major
Iliacus

*Figure 1.4: V-position, isolating the psoas major.*

As with most spine muscles, the psoas can also aid lateral bending of the lower spine (the right psoas will contract to bend the spine to the right, ipsilaterally) and contralateral rotation (the right psoas will contract to produce rotation to the left). These are very minor and weaker contractions of the psoas as compared to those in its other roles.

PART 1

Chapter 1 – Anatomy and Biomechanics of the Psoas Area

## Proximity of the Psoas Major to Other Structures

The psoas works with many other major muscles to produce and stabilize movement; these will be discussed throughout the book. Here the supporting group of lower spinal extensors will be discussed.

The **transversospinalis** muscle group is part of the deeper posterior muscles, specifically the semispinalis, multifidus, and rotatores muscles. The last two form a bundle around the lower spine with the psoas major and help straighten the spine, which is in conflict with the psoas's action of flexion of the lumbar spine. This is where practical knowledge comes into play and the *Anatomy Trains* work of Thomas Myers (2009). He explains the upper, anterior psoas fibers of the lumbar portion as appearing to help with flexion, while the lower, inner fibers help with extension. Other scientists describe the reverse. While the "jury is still out," the most important thing to keep in mind is that the psoas in an erect spine acts as a stabilizer more than a mover, with stronger spinal extensor and flexor muscles doing much of the contractional work.

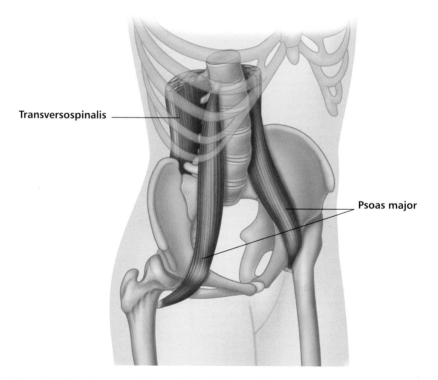

Transversospinalis

Psoas major

*Figure 1.5: The deep posterior muscles in relation to the psoas major.*

To palpate (touch) the psoas area, one would have to begin at the front of the body about 3 inches below and to the side of the naval, then travel past the abdominals, some organs, and other muscles (which is almost impossible). There in the deep core lies the psoas, one on each side of the lower spine. It is a difficult muscle to reach because of its proximity to organs, arteries, and nerves, so this is usually not advised. The muscle moves down the front of the pelvis and femur neck to attach on the lesser trochanter on the inside of the upper femur. It goes behind the **inguinal ligaments** that run from the anterior superior iliac spine (ASIS) of the pelvis to the pubic tubercle, which are both prominent points that jut out to the front of the pelvis and can be easily found. One can feel the contraction of the hip flexors by finding the lower outside rim of the ASIS and pressing there, as the thigh is lifted forward in hip flexion.

The **ilioinguinal nerve** supplies sensation to the area and must be considered in the careful treatment of the muscle, as well as the proximity of the **external iliac artery** along the medial border of the muscle. The direct continuation of the external iliac is the **femoral artery**, which supplies blood to the greater part of the lower extremity. The **genitofemoral nerve** can also be affected by closeness of the psoas and taken into account in treatment.

As mentioned before, organs can be associated with the psoas because of its central location. The **kidneys**, **ureter**, and **adrenals** are very prominent in the mid-section and must be addressed with care during therapy for the psoas.

**Fascia** covers the psoas, as it does other muscles. Fascia is a connective tissue that surrounds and separates muscle. Lumbar fascia (called lumbar **aponeurosis**) blends with psoas fascia, which extends from the first lumbar vertebra toward the sacrum, and from the crest of the ilium to the quadratus lumborum and iliacus muscles. The iliac fascia then connects and accepts the tendon of the psoas minor (if present) as well as the inguinal ligament. On toward the thigh, the psoas and iliacus fasciae form a single structure called the **iliopectineal fascia**. This fascia passes behind the femoral vessels, but the **lumbar plexus nerve** branches are posterior to it, making it an extremely complex area.

There is a large **bursa** (fluid-filled sac that provides cushioning) within the hip joint cavity. This bursa usually separates the psoas major tendon from the joint capsule and the pubis.

The positioning of the psoas in relation to the leg, pelvis, and trunk is most important. It acts as a structural conduit, guiding the support of the spine as its muscle fibers travel down and outward. However, these muscle fibers then travel back in toward the thigh, making the psoas major a **fusiform** muscle. This is a spindle-shaped muscle, wider at the middle and thinner at both ends, not unlike the biceps brachii. It appears to have an elongated trapezium shape, but must be observed three-dimensionally as it slightly spirals along with the pelvic structure it enhances.

The suspension of the psoas from the trunk to the legs helps channel movement from the spine, and aids the transfer of weight from the torso to the thighs in locomotor movements such as walking. If the psoas on one side is unbalanced with the other side, imagine what this might do to the gait or stride of a walk. If both psoas muscles (right and left sides) are healthy and can move freely, there is a steady flow to the movement and the energies that happen within the body systems.

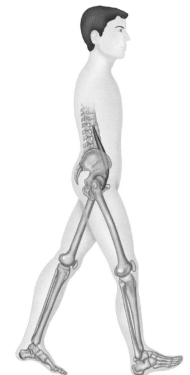

*Figure 1.6: The psoas in balance while walking.*

## The Psoas as a Major Mechanism

The psoas is considered a core muscle that acts as a keystone, central and superior to the "flying buttresses" of the femurs and thigh muscles. This major architectural concept is also apparent in the skeletal pelvis/leg relationship, and supports the human body much like an arch does in building structures.

The psoas travels vertically from the spine to the leg, and diagonally across the pelvis. As a skeletal muscle that passes across more than one joint, it becomes *bi-articulate* (a muscle that works two joints). This is a most important concept, but it is interesting to note another role of the psoas: a shelf, supporting internal organs, along with the pelvis as a basin, and the pelvic floor.

Thus, any force of the psoas (muscular contraction) can stimulate and massage organs such as the intestines, kidneys, liver, spleen, pancreas, bladder, and/or stomach. Even reproductive organs are affected. Some deep, central, internal organs are referred to as *viscera*, so communication from organs to the brain can be called *visceral messaging*. The psoas, because of its proximity to major organs, can play a role as a reactor to these stimuli, thus affecting what is commonly termed "gut feelings."

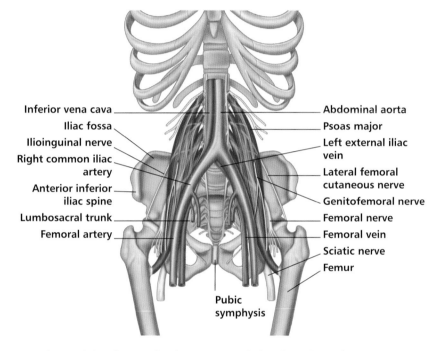

*Figure 1.7: The proximity of nerves (lumbar nerve complex) and arteries to the psoas.*

It can also affect nerve innervation, especially the **lumbar nerve complex** that passes through it. The **aorta** (the largest artery) lies in a similar path to the psoas, so body circulation and rhythms can become intertwined with the psoas as well.

Another remarkable fact is that the psoas and the **diaphragm**, a major breathing muscle, come together at a junction point known as the *solar plexus*. This is not an actual anatomical object like an organ, a bone, or a muscle; it is more an area behind the stomach, centered near the naval and in front of the aorta and diaphragm, which houses a nerve network. It is associated with the ancient chakra system and discussed in more depth in the spiritual section (Part III) of this book.

PART 1

Chapter 1 – Anatomy and Biomechanics of the Psoas Area

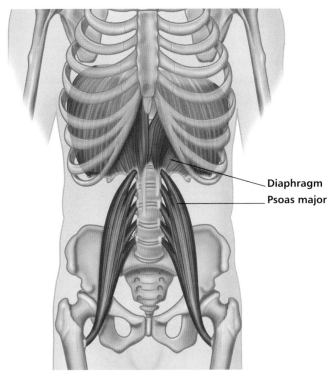

*Figure 1.8: The psoas and the diaphragm come together at a junction point known as the solar plexus.*

No wonder the psoas is so special. It has been called the "hidden prankster," the "opinionated psoas," the "great pretender," a "conductor," and the "fight or flight muscle," among other things. My wonderful physical therapist, Dr. Gary, calls it the "front butt." What a marvelous identity!

The psoas can:

- balance the core;
- stimulate organs and nerves;
- contract, release, stabilize, neutralize, or deteriorate like any other muscle;
- connect the upper body to the lower body;
- create movement and flow to be transmitted throughout the body.

It can also adapt to differences in many ways, as long as it is in a state of release (not tight or "frozen") and it is healthy. The following chapters will demonstrate how to keep the muscle in balance through various types of exercise, and discuss its role in the emotional and spiritual state of the human being.

> *The psoas affects the whole person.*

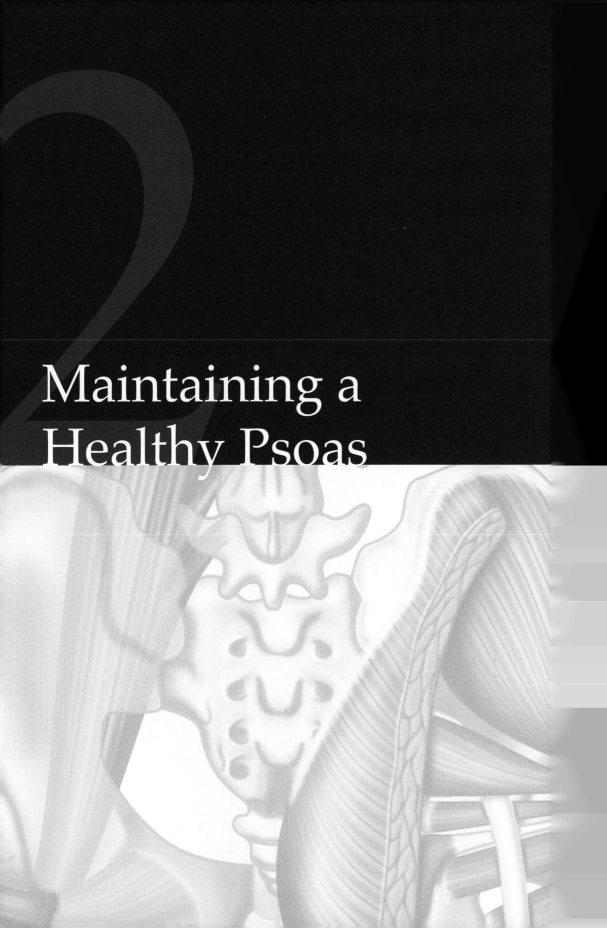

# Maintaining a
# Healthy Psoas

It has been established in Chapter 1 that the psoas major plays many roles. It is located in the core, but mostly overworked because of this. It is important to note again that other muscles have to be strong yet flexible to allow the psoas to remain healthy and adaptable. Those muscles are the abdominals, spinal extensors, and posterior antagonists such as the gluteus maximus. Any muscle that can aid in the centering and balance of the pelvis, like the quadratus lumborum and deep rotators, also helps relieve the psoas to connect the torso to the legs and act as a messenger in an economic fashion. The following exercises may help restore vitality to the psoas.

## The "Give the Psoas a Break" Exercise: Constructive Rest Position for Everyone

This is a supine position that has been taught for many years. The system was developed by Mabel Todd in the early part of the twentieth century in Boston and then in New York City as an alternative to strict military physical education. She called this method *Natural Posture*. Her ideology was later termed *Ideokinesis*, an idea of movement used to improve muscular coordination through imagery. Creative yet scientific, it is based on functional anatomy with ease and repatterning of movement, and was embraced by major universities such as Columbia, NYU, and Juilliard.

Lulu Sweigard, a student-turned-colleague of Todd's, named this certain exercise *constructive rest position* (CRP) in New York in the late 1920s. Other students, such as Barbara Clark, Sally Swift, and later Irene Dowd, became renowned teachers in the field of Ideokinesis, and people around the world have studied and embraced it as a way of rebalancing misguided physical efforts in a more natural way. This is also a concept that Joseph Pilates became aware of after the war, when he moved to New York and began work with singers and dancers; the Alexander Technique also teaches it.

Today this position is widely practiced; it is hard to find a professional dancer or body worker who has not been exposed to its benefits. This author was taught the CRP as the *horizontal rest position* at NYU many years ago, and still uses it for reasons ranging from abdominal and uteral cramping, to relaxing many muscles, specifically the psoas. It is a great way to release muscle contraction, as it allows the skeleton (and gravity) to do the work of neutral alignment in a restful state.

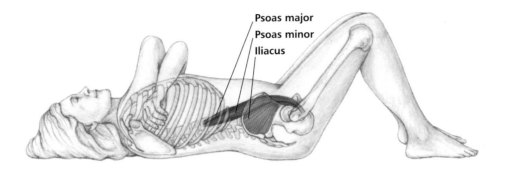

Psoas major
Psoas minor
Iliacus

*Figure 2.1: The Constructive Rest Position.*

**Technique**: Begin lying on the back (supine) on a firm, flat surface. Bend the knees with the feet flat on the floor, hip width apart. The head can be supported so that it is in line with the spine. Some prefer to keep the hips, knees, and feet in line with each other; if this is hard to do and causes muscle tension, then let the knees rest against each other with the feet slightly wider and toes turned in.

> *The femur will rest gently into the hip socket, releasing the "grip" of the hip flexors. The spine will follow its natural curves. Both arrangements free the psoas.*

Arms can be crossed at the elbows and lie across the chest; if this is uncomfortable, they can relax on the floor. (Remember, this is a rest position!)

Imagery:
1. Close the eyes and envision the full length of the spine.
2. Imagine a line of energy traveling down the spine, then curving up between the legs, moving up the front of the body and back down the spine again.
3. A cyclical energy line is engaged; inhale as it flows down the spine, exhale as it comes up the front, not unlike a "zipper being pulled up to close a jacket" around the torso.
4. Feel the weight of the head melt into the surface – not back, but in line with the neutral spine.
5. Relax and let the aligned vertebrae and pelvic bones support the body without using the muscles.
6. Feel as if the knees are draped over a hanger, the thighs hanging on one side, the lower legs on the other, with the hanger supported from above.

7. Bring mental attention to the thighs and imagine a small waterfall flowing down from the knees into the hip sockets, releasing the thigh muscles.
8. Imagine another waterfall trickling from the knees, down the shins, to the ankles. Take your time.
9. Feel the feet, as well as the eyes, relaxing in cool pools of water.
10. Repeat this full set of imagery over and over, slowly, for at least 10 minutes. When done, do not sit up, but simply roll over to one side and come to a sitting position slowly, so as not to disrupt any alignment achieved.

(This author cannot begin to remember all the wonderful teachers who taught her this strategy, but gives thanks to the mentors Andre Bernard and Irene Dowd.)

The psoas is in a relaxed state at the lumbar spine. While doing this position, it might be helpful to have someone read the imagery list slowly to help guide you. It is released at the hip; even though there is hip flexion, it is not active against resistance, so the psoas is at rest. This exercise can be done daily, anytime during the day, and by anyone, and allows the psoas to "take a break." When first practicing the technique, one may experience physical discomfort, even emotional feelings (see Part II).

> *In CRP, the body will give in to gravity — let go, and become balanced and receptive to its natural alignment and posture.*

There is another position that is very effective for releasing the psoas, as described by the *Egoscue method*, a system of exercises designed by Pete Egoscue to alleviate chronic joint pain (see bibliography). Similar in principle to the CRP, one lies on the floor with one or both lower legs resting on a block or support. The support should be as high as the length of the femur. The support holds the weight of the lower leg and allows the thigh to fall directly into the hip socket, thereby releasing the psoas and other hip and spine muscles. This position is held for as long as possible to achieve the desired relaxation. If no support is available, the feet can rest against a wall, hip width apart, with the knees bent and the hips directly underneath them. Abdominal crunches can be added without engaging the psoas too much.

# Understanding "Center": Pelvic Stability Exercises – Level I

To understand and feel the concept of a stable pelvis, try the following:

1. **Deep Breathing**: Lie on the back with knees bent, feet on the floor, hip width apart, and hands on the front hip bones to make sure they are in line with each other. Breathe naturally but deeply, engaging the transversus abdominis on a strong exhalation – one will feel as if the waist is "cinching" on the exhalation. Do this for at least five full breaths, keeping the pelvis stable.

2. **Pelvic Tilts**: Assume the same position as above, with arms by the sides. On the inhalation allow the pelvis to tilt forward; the front hip bones (ASIS) release upward, while the tailbone remains on the floor. Exhale and press the naval toward the floor as the pelvis tilts backward. Do this slowly five times, then return to normal position, which is the neutral spine curvature. The sacrum, not the lower back, will be resting on the floor, with the pelvis centered.

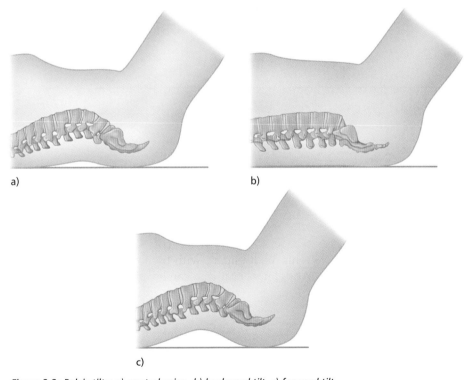

a)

b)

c)

*Figure 2.2: Pelvic tilts; a) neutral spine, b) backward tilt, c) forward tilt.*

3. **Rotational Pelvic Exercises**: Lie on the back in the position of exercise 1 with arms by the sides. Push the hips up about 2 inches off the floor, as the feet press into the floor. Try these three movements:
   a. "Hike" the hips side to side 6 times.
   b. Roll (rotate) the hips side to side 6 times.
   c. Draw a figure 8 with the hips 6 times.
      To end, roll down through the lower spine and rest the pelvis in the neutral position. One cannot help but feel where the center is after this exercise.

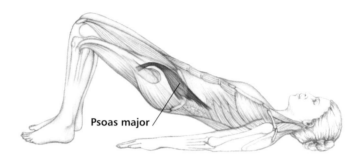

*Figure 2.3: Rotational Pelvic Exercises.*

To help visualize pelvic movement in exercises 2 and 3 above, use the reference in the following figure.

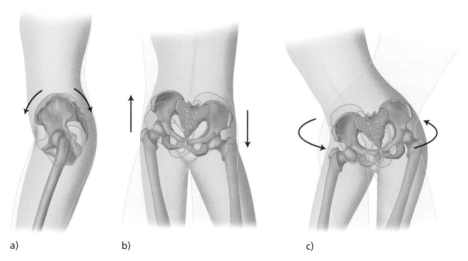

a)  b)  c)

*Figure 2.4: The pelvis can move in three planes; a) sagittal (plane 1), b) frontal (plane 2), c) horizontal (plane 3).*

**Plane 1**

In the sagittal plane, it can move forward and backward, which is usually called pelvic tilt (see figure 2.2). Use the anterior superior iliac spine (ASIS) as a reference point. This point can be felt by placing the hands on the front hip bones. Move the pelvis forward and backward. The lumbar spine will hyperextend and the hips will flex with forward movement of the pelvis. With posterior or backward tilt, the lumbar spine will flex, engaging the psoas and abdominals.

**Plane 2**

In the frontal plane, the pelvis will move laterally and medially, as in "hiking the hip up." The lumbar spine will also move laterally and the hips will abduct and adduct.

**Plane 3**

In the horizontal plane, the pelvis rotates inward and outward, although it is very limited and cannot happen without help from the sacroiliac, lumbar, and hip joints. It is similar to "twisting."

These exercises mobilize the pelvic region without overstretching. If sensitive areas such as the sacroiliac joint become too loose, the result can be irritating at the very least, and may develop into chronic lower back pain. When ligaments overstretch they do not retain their firm hold to keep the joint together, so there is a "shifting" of joint stability, and muscle tendons will work overtime to keep the joint stable. *The psoas also compensates for sacroiliac problems, which leads to it being overworked.*

To explain in more detail, the pelvis has two important joint areas: the **sacroiliac (SI) joint** and the **iliofemoral (common hip) joint**. The SI joint, where the sacrum and iliac bones (the two sides of the pelvis) articulate, is the least moveable. It is considered a gliding joint and becomes more active during childbirth.

There are strong **ligaments** that connect the iliac bones to the sacrum. Therefore, it seems reasonable to assume that many women after childbirth can experience a sacroiliac shift because of loosened ligaments. This can cause discomfort in the lower back area that can be addressed through some strength exercises to compensate for the laxity. The squat exercise described on page 28 is an ideal strength move for this area if done in the position of outward rotation of the hip. Grand plies from ballet are also helpful.

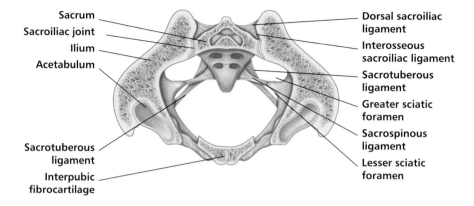

Sacrum
Sacroiliac joint
Ilium
Acetabulum

Dorsal sacroiliac ligament
Interosseous sacroiliac ligament
Sacrotuberous ligament
Greater sciatic foramen
Sacrospinous ligament

Sacrotuberous ligament
Interpubic fibrocartilage

Lesser sciatic foramen

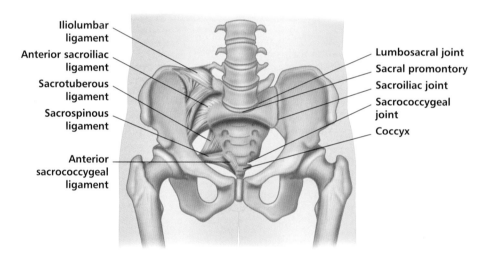

Iliolumbar ligament
Anterior sacroiliac ligament
Sacrotuberous ligament
Sacrospinous ligament
Anterior sacrococcygeal ligament

Lumbosacral joint
Sacral promontory
Sacroiliac joint
Sacrococcygeal joint
Coccyx

*Figure 2.5: The sacroiliac joint; a) transverse section of the pelvis, b) pelvic ligaments.*

The six deep outward rotators of the hip are small **muscles** that can be targeted for help with stability at the SI joint, as they travel from the sacrum, across the pelvis to the femur. These include the **piriformis**, two **gemelli**, two **obturators**, and the **quadratus femoris**. View figure 2.6 and notice the positioning of the sciatic nerve behind the piriformis. If the muscle is too contracted, it will pinch the nerve and become a major factor in "sciatica." The SI stretch on page 31 will alleviate this pressure.

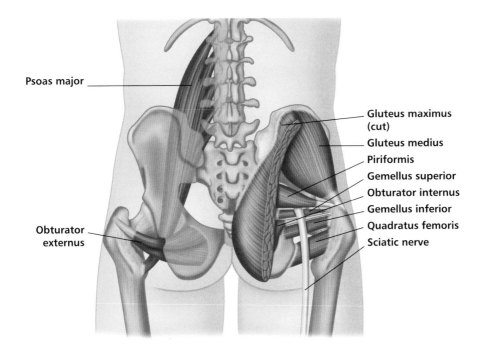

*Figure 2.6: The six deep outward rotators.*

## Sacroiliac Joint Exercises

Exercises that incorporate the abdominals, erector spinae, gluteus maximus, and deep external rotators of the hip to engage properly will help the sacroiliac joint remain strong yet supple, like the psoas should be. These can be done complementary to pelvic stability exercises.

1. **Squats** (Level I/II): There are many myths about squats, and most people would not consider them an exercise for the SI joint. Done properly and without extreme resistance, they can achieve great results for pelvic, core, and hip strength, developing protection for the SI joint and psoas.

**Technique**:
   a. Begin standing in front of a mirror with a chair behind.
   b. Hold a lightweight bar or band above the head without lifting the shoulders. The latissimus dorsi, fascia, and ribs will stretch away from the pelvis.
   c. Engage the abdominals and erector spinae muscles as the knees bend to lower to a sitting position.
   d. Allow the hips to fall back toward the chair, and bend deeply at the hips. Keep the head and chest forward without expanding the rib cage. If the upper thighs can come parallel to the floor, it is most effective.
   e. Hold the sitting position for 10–20 seconds. The gluteus maximus, as well as the core, will work here and on the way back up from this position.

Repeat the exercise 5–10 times, stretching the body up and slightly back in between each repetition to open the front of the hips. Do not lose the engagement of the core and gluteus maximus, or hyperextend the lower back, while stretching.

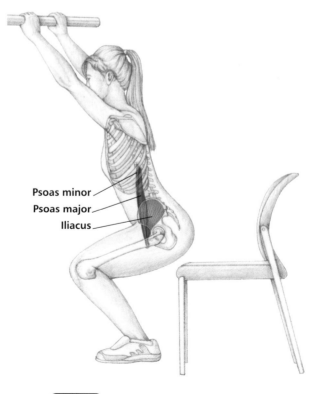

Psoas minor
Psoas major
Iliacus

*Figure 2.7: Squats.*

2. **Spinal Twists** (Level I): Standing spinal twists are the most beneficial rotation exercises when the gluteus maximus also needs to be targeted.

**Technique**: Stand straight with feet hip width apart. Keep the pelvis forward and rotate the upper spine (thoracic and cervical) to the right, as the gluteus maximus is squeezed and the core engaged (do not overdo it – this can be a gentle contraction). Elongate the spine and breath deeply as the twist is held. The hips can twist slightly; this will protect the lower spine, SI joint, and psoas. Repeat on the other side.

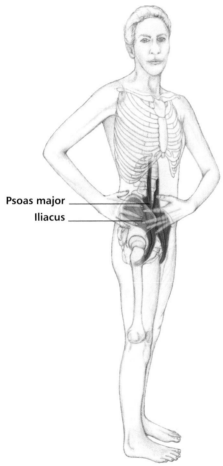

Psoas major _____

Iliacus _____

*Figure 2.8: Spinal Twists.*

3. **Hand/Knee Balance** (Level I/II)

**Technique**: Assume the table position ("all fours"), making sure the hands are under the shoulders and the knees are under the hips.

**Level I**: Stretch one leg behind, to hip height, and release the opposite arm forward. The pelvis remains centered with the core engaged.

**Level II**: Assume the position above, but with the support hand and knee in line with each other. This will narrow the base and challenge the balance. Hold for 10–20 seconds. Add a "sit-back," releasing the gluteus maximus back toward the heel and hold for added benefit.

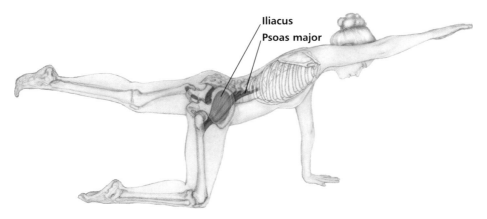

*Figure 2.9: Hand/Knee Balance.*

4. **SI Stretch** (Level I): If this area is too tight, it can be slowly stretched with the following exercise. The upper psoas is also affected, while the distal psoas is released. This is also a great stretch for the iliotibial band and smaller glutes.

**Technique**: Lie on the back with the legs straight and the arms outstretched. Bend one knee toward the chest and let it fall to the opposite side; allow the hips to roll with it. Keep the shoulders on the floor, but do not push them. Breathe and relax; never force a twist. Repeat with the other leg.

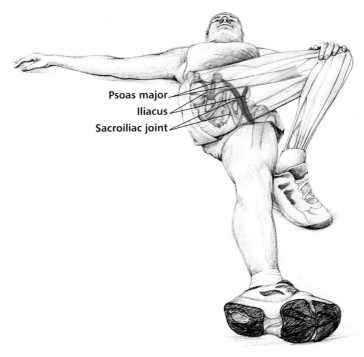

Psoas major
Iliacus
Sacroiliac joint

*Figure 2.10: Sacroiliac Joint Stretch.*

## Finding Balance: Upright Stability Exercises

The psoas acts in a sense like a pendulum, allowing the swing of the heavy leg forward from the spine to walk. Knowing this, it is of paramount importance that *the pelvis remains centered in its placement as the psoas connects to the movement*. Of course, the pelvis will mobilize slightly but remain the central hub while going "with" the movement.

The pelvis is two-sided, with the sacrum in the middle; both sides need to be in balance with each other. Major stabilizing muscles like the **quadratus lumborum** and **transversus abdominis** can be engaged to allow the pelvis to be centered and the psoas to be free to aid transfer of weight in upright movement.

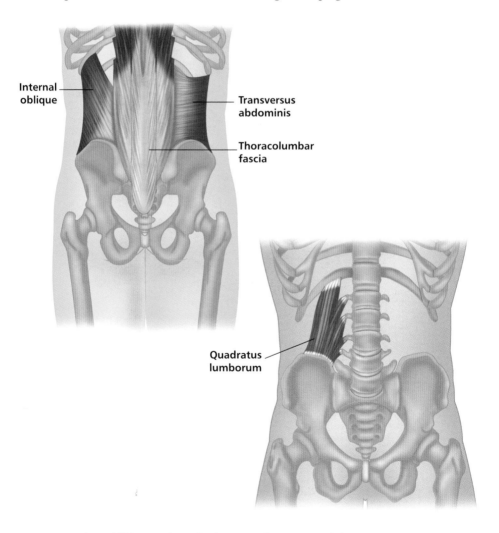

Internal oblique

Transversus abdominis

Thoracolumbar fascia

Quadratus lumborum

*Figure 2.11: The stabilizing quadratus lumborum and transversus abdominis.*

1. **Walk Without Wiggling** (Level I): It is hard to keep from swaying the hips sideways (laterally). Keep the pelvis centered and allow the legs to move freely, otherwise the psoas will be overworked. The pelvis will rotate minimally with alternately one side forward and the other side back. Allow this to happen as the leg swings forward.

2. **One-Leg Balances** (Level II): There are many of these to choose from – try the following:

    a. **Ballet barre exercises** such as the passé position.

**Technique**: Stand on one leg and take the other one to passé position (bent knee, outward rotated hip, foot pointed to inside of standing knee). Keeping hips level, one can remain balanced while strengthening the legs and core. To increase strength, hold on to the barre or a wall and develop the supporting leg by doing pliés and relevés (bending the knee, then rising to the ball of the foot). Always track the knee over the toes.

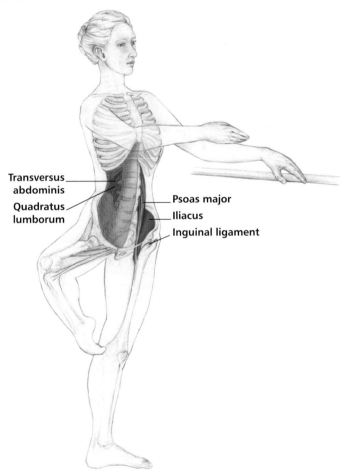

*Figure 2.12: Standing postures for balance, support, and alignment for the ballet barre.*

b. **Yoga postures** such as Tree Pose.

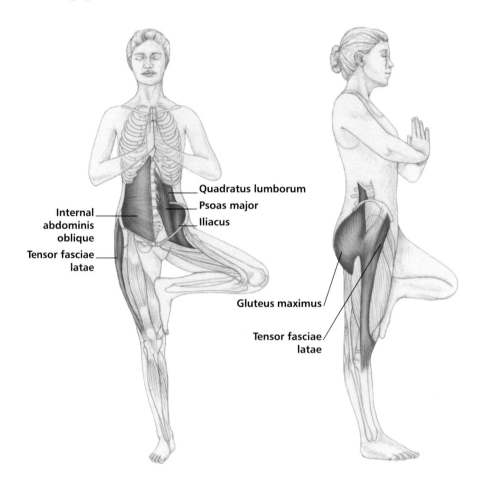

*Figure 2.13: Tree Pose.*

In each of the one-leg standing exercises, use the pelvis centrally without hiking the hip up with the higher leg. Extend the spine, drop the tailbone, and lift the abdominals, not the shoulders. Relax the rib cage. This pattern will correct most misalignment issues.

Observe the body in a mirror to help correct any imbalance. The supporting side is strengthening isometrically, while the free leg is both strengthening and stretching. The psoas is working differently on each side, so balancing the pelvis will aid the necessary mechanics needed to stabilize, strengthen, and/or stretch.

## Stimulating the Pelvic Floor: Balls and the Kegel

The pelvic floor is an area of deep, lower muscles near the base of the spine, where a sheet sometimes referred to as the urogenital diaphragm lies with other muscles such as the sphincter, bulbospongiosus, and perinea. These muscles have important functions during breathing, sex, and childbirth, and are a center for sensitive nerve endings, as is the psoas. When stimulated and strengthened, the area can influence energy, sensations, and emotions. Organs like the bladder and kidneys are also affected.

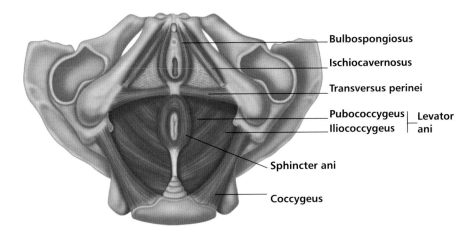

*Figure 2.14: The pelvic floor muscles.*

One of the best ways to develop this deep center correctly is by doing the following exercises:

1. **Ball Therapy** (Level I): A great exercise after sitting for long periods of time!
   a. Lie down with small exercise balls (4–6 inches in diameter) under the pelvis, around the lower buttocks. Bend the knees with the feet flat on the floor. The pressure of the balls allows the organs to shift upward, releasing stress away from the pelvic floor. The person can then lift one or both legs, as in the Happy Baby Pose from yoga (see Part III), to center and strengthen the area. In Happy Baby, supine position, the knees are bent and separated with the thighs against the lateral ribs; the hands can hold the feet, which are parallel to the ceiling. For lower abdominal and pelvic floor strength, try lifting the hips straight up off the balls, repeating 5–10 times.

Raising and lowering one leg at a time from a straight leg position will incorporate psoas work, if needed, by both strengthening and stretching, making the psoas elastic and responsive. Finish with both legs straight on the floor with the spine relaxed in neutral position to open the front of the hips.

b. For core stability, change the position of the balls so that one is a bit higher on the hip, on the sacroiliac joint. Place the other ball on the opposite side of the mid back on the erector spinae, about an inch away from the spine. Begin to "balance the core" by keeping weight into the balls even; repeat on the other side. This can be done with legs bent, feet flat on the floor.

*Once pelvic movement versus stability is experienced, a pattern of alignment that emphasizes correct mechanics to aid the psoas can be developed.*

2. **The Kegel**: Named after the gynecologist Dr. Arnold Kegel, the movement strengthens pelvic floor muscles.

**Technique**: This can be done lying down, sitting, or standing: simply put, squeeze the sit bones together, and hold and breathe. This lifts the pelvic floor and stimulates the entire area, improving muscle tone. It is used to prepare for childbirth and to aid incontinence and sexual function. The relation to the psoas is balance and support by strengthening the muscles around it. While squeezing sit bones towards one another, do not contract the larger muscles such as the gluteus maximus and abdominals – smaller muscles including the ones that control urine flow need to be activated to incorporate the pelvic floor.

"Lifting the pelvic floor" is a cue that can be used to help stabilize the core, as long as it is described so the client can understand it. Phrases such as "hugging the lower abdominals" are effective and can create the upward movement needed. This affects the connection of the pelvic floor, transversus abdominis, psoas major and diaphragm in a balanced and unique way.

# Core Strengthening Exercises

Almost any core exercise to strengthen the area will include the psoas. The most important thing to remember is that the psoas is probably already overworked, so other core muscles must be emphasized.

1. **Side-Bending** (Level I)

**Technique:** Stand with feet shoulder-width apart. Keep body upright and bend to the left or to the right. Can be performed sitting, kneeling, or standing, and is both a strength and stretch exercise for the abdominals. Arms overhead will add difficulty.

*Main movers*: Spinal extensors. Abdominals.
*Inner core stabilizers*: Quadratus lumborum. Psoas.

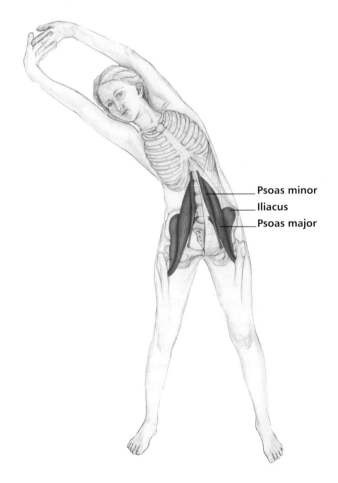

Psoas minor
Iliacus
Psoas major

*Figure 2.15: Side-Bending.*

2. **Partial Sit-up** (Levels I–II)

**Technique**: Lie on back (supine position) with knees bent, and feet on the floor. Flex the spine (always exhale when flexing), coming up halfway, and roll back down through each vertebra on the inhale.

*Main movers*: Rectus abdominis.
*Inner core stabilizers*: Psoas. Pelvic floor.

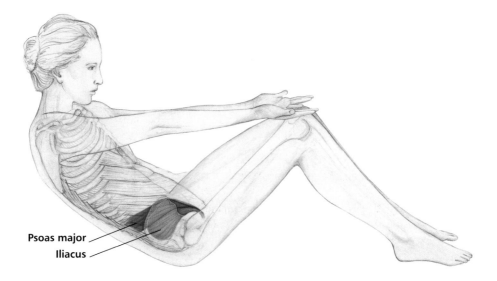

Psoas major
Iliacus

*Figure 2.16: Partial Sit-Up.*

3. **Windmills** (Level I)

**Technique**: Standing with arms out to sides, touch right hand to left ankle, stand up and repeat to other side. This will do all three actions of the external oblique, and provide both a strength and stretch exercise. It is mild because rotation is minimal against resistance – bend knees slightly to keep from hyperextending them.

*Main movers*: Internal and external obliques. Spinal rotators/extensors.
*Inner core stabilizers*: Quadratus lumborum. Psoas. Transversospinalis group.

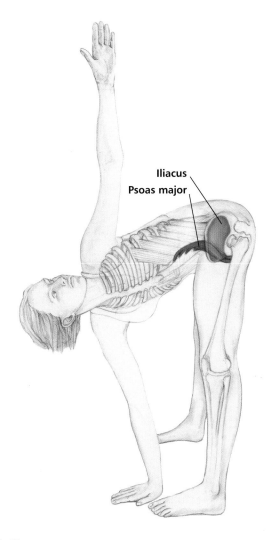

*Figure 2.17: Windmills.*

### 4. Roman Chair Rotational Crunches

**Technique**: (This exercise is very hard on the lumbar (lower) spine, so make sure that the abdominals are strong to begin with.) Sit sideways on a bench with feet stabilized on the floor. Lie back slowly in a curled (flexed) position until parallel with the floor; return. To isolate the obliques, rotate the spine, alternating sides on the return.

*Main movers*: Rectus abdominis. Hip flexors.
*Inner core stabilizers*: Psoas. Pelvic floor.

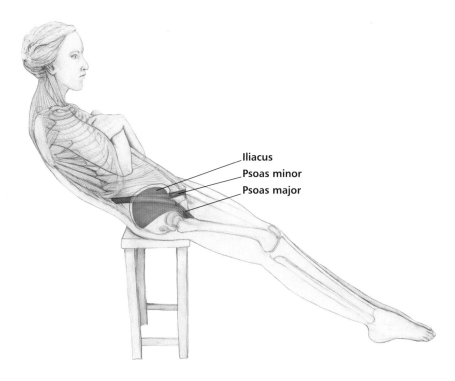

Iliacus
Psoas minor
Psoas major

*Figure 2.18: Roman Chair Rotational Crunches.*

### 5. Hip Rolls

**Technique**: Lie on back, knees into chest and arms out to sides in 'T' position, palms down. Rolls knees to one side, then the other.

Do this at least five times; inhale on the way down, exhale back up to center, engaging the core. If there is back pain, do not allow the legs to go all the way to the floor.

*Main movers*: Obliques.
*Inner core stabilizers*: Transverse abdominis. Psoas.

## Stretching Exercises

Since the psoas has so many attachments and roles, it is confusing to know when and where it needs to be stretched. The most important rule is: **if there is a lot of time spent sitting, the lower psoas is relaxed in a shortened state, and needs to lengthen and open to counteract sitting hip flexion**. The following exercises will accomplish this.

1. **Rising Stomach Stretch** (Level I): The abdominals must be engaged in this exercise so as not to injure the lower spine.

**Technique**: Lie face down and bring the hands close to the shoulders. Keep the hips on the ground, look forward and rise up by straightening the arms. If there is back pain, do not straighten the arms completely, and always press the shoulders down away from the ears.

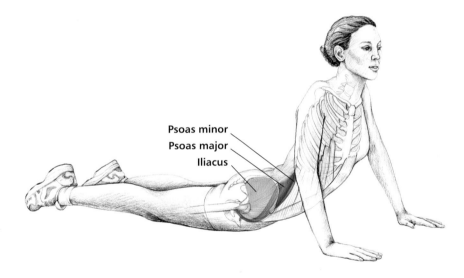

Psoas minor
Psoas major
Iliacus

*Figure 2.19: Rising Stomach Stretch.*

2. **Half Bridge** (Level I)

**Technique**: Lying on back with knees bent and feet flat on floor, curl the tailbone off the floor; begin to raise hips as high as what feels comfortable. Weight should be evenly distributed to both feet and shoulder blades. If there is discomfort in the sacroiliac area, keep the supporting leg straight while lifting the hip.

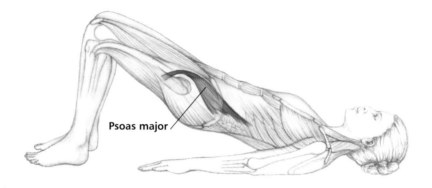

*Figure 2.20: Half Bridge.*

3. **Psoas Lift** (Level I)

**Technique**: Lie on floor with knees bent, feet on floor shoulder-width apart, and arms out for support. Move right leg to one side while feet remain on floor. Lift left hip off the floor and hold the stretch. Repeat on the other side. If there is discomfort in the sacroiliac area, keep the supporting leg straight while lifting the hip.

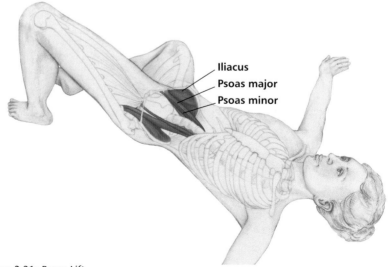

*Figure 2.21: Psoas Lift.*

4. **Lunges (Runner's Stretch)** (Level I / II)

**Technique**: Begin standing with the left foot forward and the right leg back. Bend the front knee until it is directly over the toes; slide the right leg straight back until it is parallel to the floor, if possible. Keep the feet facing forward and do not let the front knee go farther forward than the toes. The spine is straight and the hands can rest on the floor or the front thigh. *The hip flexors are strengthening in the front leg and stretching in the back leg.* Hold for approximately 30 seconds, then repeat on the other side.

**Variation**: Push the hips forward and drop the back knee to the floor to increase the stretch of the psoas. Deepen the stretch by sliding the right leg back further with the heel off the ground.

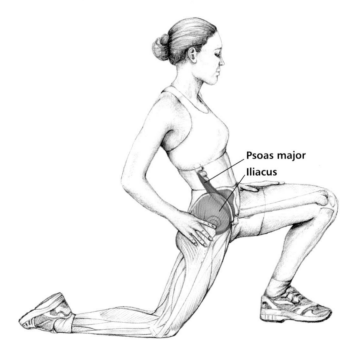

Psoas major
Iliacus

*Figure 2.22: Variations of Lunges (Runner's Stretch).*

*See Chapter 4 in this part for Pilates, and Part III for yoga exercises that will also strengthen or stretch the psoas area.*

## Review: Fact or Fiction?

### The psoas is a muscle.
Fact – it was probably one of the first skeletal muscles. When talking about the psoas, it is important to remember that it is the psoas major muscle of the iliopsoas muscle group that is usually indicated.

### The psoas causes back pain.
Fact – there can, however, be other reasons for back pain, and the psoas is not usually the main culprit.

### The psoas is not a hip flexor.
Fiction – still under debate, its role as a hip flexor is not a major one, but, as part of the iliopsoas muscle group and because of its path, the psoas can aid in the action of hip flexion, depending on the movement.

### The psoas is part of the core.
Fact – it is part of the deeper core, as it attaches to the transverse process of the lumbar spinal column and travels anteriorly past the pelvis.

### The psoas cannot be palpated.
Fiction – it can be touched, but at the cost of disturbing other structures and stimulating the involuntary response of "fight or flight."

### The psoas moves in all three planes.
Fact – it can minimally contract or stretch in the sagittal, frontal, and horizontal planes, but is mostly a sagittal-plane muscle.

### The psoas works alone.
Fiction – it is in fact extremely hard to isolate, as its action is synergistic with many other muscles.

### The psoas can be stretched.
Fact – at the hip, any position that places the thigh behind the pelvis is a stretch for the lower psoas on that side.

### The psoas is a mover more than a stabilizer.
Fiction – at the lumbar spine, and also as it travels to the femur, the psoas becomes more important as a stabilizer and postural muscle.

The psoas is the only muscle that connects the upper and lower extremities. Fact!

# 3

# The Strain of Lower Back Pain

The lower (lumbar) spine is an elaborate system of nerves, bones, muscles, ligaments, and other tissues that combine to create one of the most abused areas of the body. In the United States alone, lower back pain has become a "disease" of unknown proportions, causing an infinite number of insurance claims, unemployment, and disability, resulting in a loss of billions of dollars each year. It can be either acute (short term) or *chronically progressive*, with symptoms ranging from soreness to an inability to stand up and move.

## Anatomy of the Lumbar Area

The lumbar spine has the same functions as the rest of the spine: support, mobility, connection, balance, and protection. The differences lie in its location and size. The lumbar area supports the weight of the upper extremity. The vertebrae are larger and thicker to help accomplish this, but this can also limit movement. It is also an integral part of the core.

There are five lumbar vertebrae, approximately located in the center of the body. Because they are larger and thicker than the other bones of the spine, they are also heavier. They have a *lordotic* curve, meaning anterior curve or toward the front, which counterbalances the thoracic posterior curve. The *discs* (the cartilage in between the bones) are one-third the thickness of the vertebral bodies, which allows for mobility in flexion, extension, and lateral bending; but rotation is limited due to the straight projection, short length, and bulky properties of the posterior spinal processes, along with the orientation of the facets (articulating surfaces of a vertebra process).

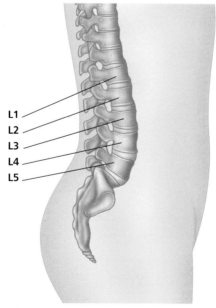

L1
L2
L3
L4
L5

*Figure 3.1: The lumbar spine.*

As seen in previous illustrations, the psoas is also centrally located here, with attachments to the lateral lumbar processes. Therefore, *the psoas becomes one of the main muscles that can affect the condition of the lower back* as well as the positioning of the pelvis. Both the lower spine and the pelvis are interdependent: they must be in balance and alignment with each other to function properly. Any incongruence will affect other areas, from the upper spine to the feet, and even cause tension in the jaw. Essentially the entire length of the body is affected, but especially the lower back.

The causes of lower back pain can be difficult to determine in each individual. The following is a list of the more common sources of pain:

- Poor posture
- Weak muscle strength (abdominals, psoas, spinal erectors)
- Hereditary conditions
- Sudden injury
- Vertebral disc problems
- Aging
- Being overweight
- Nerve disorders

Although all ages and nationalities and both genders can be affected, the primary group targeted is aged between 30 and 60. Much research has been done to explain the reasons for such widespread lumbar distress, with results showing that increasingly sedentary lifestyles, coupled with intermittent vigorous exercise, is a strong culprit.

## Psoas and Pelvic Floor Exercises to Aid the Lower Back

This is a 10-minute Level I routine (depending on injury) for the lower back. All exercises are performed in a supine position on the floor and can be done daily.

Warm-up: Lie on the back, with the knees bent and feet on the floor. Breathing deeply, engage the transversus abdominis on a strong exhale (by "cinching the waist"), to stabilize the lower spine/pelvis.

1. Pelvic Tilts: Tilt the pelvis forward and back, 5 times slowly (page 23).
2. Stretch: Lie on the back and pull the knees to the chest – hold for up to 1 minute, breathing deeply.*
3. Stretch: Cross one ankle over the other bent knee and roll the legs side to side 5 times, with arms out to the sides. Switch legs and repeat. See a variation on page 31.

*Breath work is important – a private session with a qualified instructor will aid in this, and also provide cueing to correct any misalignment or misuse.*

4. Spine Articulation: Half Bridge (page 42). Squeeze the sit bones together (Kegel) for added work at the end, before rolling down the spine.
5. Spine Stabilization and Strength: This exercise incorporates psoas and hip flexor work. Lie on the back, and raise one leg (no more than 12 inches) and lower 5 times. Keep the spine and abdominals lengthened, and the pelvis stable. Repeat with the other leg. Never do both legs together – it puts too much strain on the lower back. You may turn over and do the same thing in the prone position, making sure that the core is engaged.
6. Crossed Leg Stretch: This stretch is for the sacroiliac joint, piriformis, and other lower back muscles. Lie on the back, and cross one knee over the other (thighs together). Roll slowly to the opposite side of the top leg and hold for approximately 10 seconds, then roll to the other side and hold for 10 seconds. Switch legs and repeat.

Cool-down: Constructive Rest Position (pages 20–22).

## Causes of Back Pain: Scenarios

### Scenario 1: The Weekend Athlete

Most people in this category will have trouble admitting it. No one wants to confess that they are no longer serious athletes who used to spend almost every day of the week training.

Whether a student or a professional, there are millions of people who are spending more time sitting and less time moving. Time is a consideration, as the stress of everyday living such as working, raising a family, commuting, and studying (to name a few), takes away precious moments that could also include taking care of one's health.

Time management is important, and the lack of it has spawned a new industry of courses, videos, and the like to help advise and teach usually intelligent people how to handle their daily lives. We are all guilty, as we allow many things to get in the way of our own health. Consideration for the physical condition of the body cannot be overlooked for long, as injuries such as lower back pain will result.

### Scenario 2: Children

By now most people are aware of a growing trend of more obese children. In the United States, a country where so much is made available to a majority of the population, incorrect eating habits and sitting too much have affected our children's health.

As first lady, in 2009, Michele Obama chose this one problem for the main focus of her time in the White House through the "Let's Move" program. Uniting parents, children, teachers, leaders, and medical professionals, it is hoped that through community effort and national attention this epidemic will be curbed. Physical activity needs to be included in the process, as being overweight can and will affect the lower back, among other things.

## Scenario 3: The Overachiever

This is the opposite of the above two situations as far as movement is concerned. For purposes of this book, the *overachiever* is the physical "nut" – the one who overtrains. The body's example of "type A," this person does not know when to stop. He/she might exercise every day, for hours. The body fatigues but this person keeps going, which affects the very physiology of the joints and muscles. They can be overloaded to the extreme, without taking in enough nutrients needed to keep them working properly.

Hence the following story.

# Psoas Story: The Case of the Elusive Six-Pack ABS

**Dr. Gary Mascilak, D.C., P.T., C.S.C.S.***

Dr. W is a 28-year-old male who was presented to my office with lower back pain. Studies show that more than 8.5 out of 10 people, at some point in their lives, will have an episode of back pain that causes them to alter their daily functions.

The challenge for clinicians is always to determine the *cause* of their patient's symptoms. It is quite like detective work: I look for clues in the way they walk into my office, how they sit when I am talking with them, how they move their torso in various directions, and especially how they squat. Mobility of the hips, flexibility of the lower extremity musculature, and core strength are just a few areas that are critical to assess.

The most important component of a clinician's examination is taking a thorough history. Dr. W seemed somewhat agitated during this process, and I did not think his reaction was merely from pain. When I politely inquired if he was very uncomfortable, he said he was more frustrated because he had not been able to do his "normal" things for over two

*Dr. Gary Mascilak is the clinic director and co-owner of Integrated Health Professionals, a multi-disciplinary rehabilitation center in Sparta, New Jersey. He is a licensed doctor of chiropractic, physical therapist, certified strength and conditioning specialist, and board eligible diplomate in orthopedics. He has been in practice for over 23 years, treating a variety of orthopedic and sports injuries, from professional to adolescent athletes and everything in between. He has lectured nationally on rehabilitation techniques and has contributed articles to professional journals and magazines, including* Runner's World *and* Sports Illustrated.

weeks. He looked very fit, so I asked him if exercising was one of the things he could not do as of late, *since individuals who routinely work out and then have to stop for one reason or another are chemically deprived of their natural opiate and endorphin "feel good" chemicals*, and can get somewhat "cranky."

Also having sensed that Dr. W may be a Type A person, I thought it was imperative that I understand what his workout entailed, as incorrect performance of exercise or excessive volume of a particular exercise can often be the culprit for the development of muscle imbalances and subsequent symptomatology. When Dr. W reported doing 1,000 sit-ups a day (2 sets of 500), I knew we had discovered a key component to his pain. Examination ultimately revealed lumbar facet syndrome, a condition where the joints of the lower back become compressed and irritated. The normal concave arch (lordosis) in his lower back was accentuated and excessive. Evaluation revealed marked hip flexor tightness on both sides, and *exquisite tenderness to palpation of the psoas muscle bilaterally*. Additionally, the exam revealed significant lower abdominal and gluteus maximus weakness, which should not be the case with someone working out for almost two hours a day, five times a week. He provided me with the exercises he was doing, and when asked to describe one of the 1,000 sit-ups he was performing each day, he indicated a basic crunch move.

Dr. W's exercises were far from a balanced routine and definitely not specific to address his existing muscle imbalances, which actually caused his repetitive injury. *His crunch exercise, as is so commonly performed, was utilizing primarily his hip flexors to perform the movement, compensating for weak abdominals*. Although crunches can be performed with proper instruction, good form, and knowledge about how to properly set the core musculature (including the pelvic floor and lower abdominals – transversus abdominis), I prefer to train the abdominal wall with different types of exercise that allow proper recruitment of the aforementioned stabilizing muscles, and *prevent* hip flexor and psoas hyperactivity and compensation.

The reverse crunch is preferred to the standard crunch as it makes the person bring the knees maximally to the chest, thereby placing the psoas in a position where it is helping flex the hip, and does not aid the abdominal muscles much to perform actions at the spine (the movement of drawing the knees to the chest and lifting the lower spine off the floor). Proper instruction is obviously still required and form needs to be monitored until mastered.

Release of hip flexors was done with soft tissue work on Dr. W, and he was instructed in proper psoas stretching exercises in all three planes of motion. Additionally, he was given exercises and instruction in strengthening his gluteal, lower abdominal, and other core muscles.

In three to four weeks, these exercises reduced the excessive arch in Dr. W's back and relieved his back pain. As a physician who attempted to treat himself for over a month with no real improvement, Dr. W inquired how I came to the conclusion as to the cause of his symptoms so rapidly. I told him that after logically examining all the clues for his case, especially his history, ultimately deducing the improper performance of the sit-ups was quite elementary (and no . . . Dr. W's last name was not Watson).

There are more scenarios, to be sure, but the above three are widespread. Exercises and/or positions to alleviate lower back pain can be found throughout this book. The appendix, "The Hip Flexion Society," will also be an invaluable aid.

The following chapter will address the more specific conditioning program of Pilates and how it works the psoas and lower back (to excess if done incorrectly).

The most important thing to remember in any exercise program is:

*Muscle balance is key to a healthy body.*

# Review: Fact or Fiction?

## Lower back pain is a disease.
Fact – it is a specific disorder that can become a medical condition affecting many people, and is therefore a disease.

## The lumbar spine is the lower back.
Fact – there are five lumbar vertebrae that, as a single area, curve anteriorly and make up the main length of what is called the lower back.

## The lumbar spine is considered small.
Fiction – although it comprises only five vertebrae, the vertebral bodies are the largest and heaviest in comparison to the rest of the spinal column.

## The lumbar spine can move in all three planes.
Fact – this is true of all mobile sections of the spine, yet each area has its limitations. At the lumbar spine, rotation is minimal because of the characteristics of its bony processes and facets.

## Rotation as a joint action of the lumbar area should be forced.
Fiction – since the action of rotation is minimal in the lower back because of bone configuration, any forceful movement beyond normal can be detrimental. (Yoga teachers and students: beware of spinal twisting in this area!)

## Lordosis is a disease.
Fiction – lordosis is the term used to indicate a concave, or anterior curve, in the spinal column, which is the correct curvature for the lumbar and cervical areas. If the lordotic curve is advanced, it can create problems, but the term itself indicates the normal position.

## The psoas major and the lumbar spine are connected.
Fact – tendons of the proximal psoas are attached to all five lumbar vertebrae.

## The psoas is considered an abdominal muscle.
Fiction – along with the quadratus lumborum, it makes up the posterior abdominal wall, but is not one of the four primary abdominals.

## The psoas is one of the main muscles affecting the lower back.
Fact – since it is located and attached here, its condition warrants attention in lower back pain.

## Sitting can cause lower back problems.
Fact! – See the appendix on "the hip flexion society."

# 4

## The Psoas and Pilates

A full chapter is devoted to Pilates, as it has become a popular and successful conditioning program. If teaching is done correctly, a certified Pilates instructor can effectively lead a person or class through a workout with attention paid to injury prevention, correct body placement, and focused muscle work. The psoas is very involved, sometimes to a fault. The instructor must cue the student properly, explaining the neutral spinal curves and not forcing the flattening of the lower back into the surface. *Using "naval to spine" is only an image that helps engage the abdominals and psoas to fall toward the spine, then lengthen; compression is not the goal.* **If the core is forced into its depths, there will be no freedom of movement. It takes practice to find the necessary quality of motion that allows flow without restriction. It is a lifelong process.**

## Why Pilates?

A Pilates workout is based on concepts of body alignment (in general posture as well as during the exercises), muscle balance or lack thereof, strength, and flexibility: all areas the psoas is a component of, depending on the movement. This section will concentrate on the mechanical role of the psoas in relation to specific "classical" Pilates mat exercises.

Almost all Pilates work includes hip and spinal flexion/extension, which the psoas can be part of, not solely, but integrally. It is known as a hip flexor because it is connected with the iliopsoas muscle group, and has a lumbar spine attachment, where its role is still debated. But the psoas is mostly involved in Pilates work because of its link from the upper to the lower extremity. This makes it a central core muscle along with the abdominals, quadratus lumborum, and other spinal extensors; but it is the only one to connect to the leg. In all exercises these muscles must help each other do their jobs in relation to body movement and positioning. If the psoas has to be the only stabilizer, it will not be released enough to be receptive. When the pelvis is stable, the psoas can go about its "business."

Pilates is an excellent workout program, with minimal drawbacks: biomechanically, there is a lot of hip flexion, and not as much stretch as most people believe. However, there is "length" presented in every exercise, which can compensate for this. There is also the possibility of *too much* core work. Overworked muscles tend to be tight, and the core needs to breathe.

Cueing the breath is essential in every exercise, as well as knowing the basic principles of mind/muscle control, a stable center, balanced flow, kinesthetic awareness, and moving without tension. Muscle endurance as well as strength is optimized when one does Pilates correctly, with precision and commitment. Find a Pilates instructor who understands this approach and has in-depth knowledge of the human body, without forcing the body into injury.

## The Classical Beginner Pilates Mat Routine: Moving without Tension

Listed in order of presentation during a class, the following exercises indicate psoas work. Keep in mind, most Pilates floor exercises (except the Hundred) are repeated five or six times, with slower, controlled motion the emphasis.

1. **The Hundred**: The psoas is strengthened minimally as both a hip and lumbar spine flexor, and a lower spine extensor, so it is one of the muscles engaged in this exercise. When the legs are straight, at a 90-degree angle, and the pelvis is fixed, the psoas helps stabilize the spine as well as work secondarily with the iliacus as the legs lower to 45 degrees. During the exercise the psoas also flexes the upper lumbar spine, along with the abdominals, and stabilizes the flexed position while the arms beat 100 times. Care should be taken not to flex the lower lumbar region, as the spine remains neutral.

   The Hundred can begin as a Level I exercise if the knees are bent, and then be increased to the Level II version explained above (legs at 45 degrees).

**Technique**: Lie on back, then flex the spine with the feet either on or off the floor, knees bent (legs straight and/or lowered is more advanced); the position is held, and the "100" is how many times the arms pump (arms are held straight in at the sides of the body). This position also strengthens the anterior neck muscles.

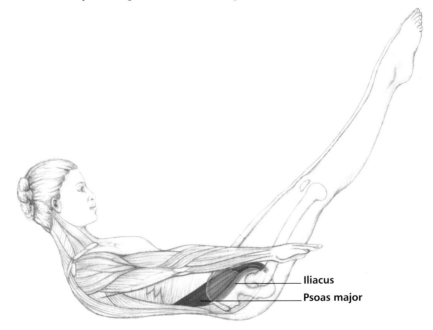

Iliacus

Psoas major

*Figure 4.1: The Pilates Hundred, Level II.*

2. **The Roll-Up**: Another good psoas worker, the Roll-Up causes the psoas to contract harder during the second half of the exercise, when the abdominals begin to work less against gravity as the body lifts into more hip and spine flexion. There is a moment when the psoas sits back against the spine as it responds to the movement.

   The Roll-Up is usually done at the beginning of a basic Pilates class, but after teaching for many years, this author feels a straight leg Roll-Up with arms reaching toward the front is actually an intermediate movement for many people. Begin with the knees bent, heels on the floor, and hands connected to the floor to aid the lower back and increase muscle awareness by allowing both sides of the body (and psoas!) to work equally as one rolls up. The roll back down is just as important.

   If this is too easy and the back responds well, then the regular Roll-Up can be done with straight legs.

   The illustration shows Level II, which can be accomplished only if the abdominals, psoas, and integral muscles are strong enough.

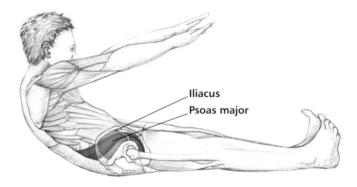

*Figure 4.2: The Roll-Up, Level II. Press shoulders down and back as the arms reach forward.*

> *Given that the psoas muscles are responsible for so much, they can actually become overworked and too fatigued. The most important concept to remember is that the psoas needs to function correctly in all its roles, without limiting it to strength and tightness.*

3.  **Single Leg Circles**: This one is interesting from a psoas point of view. The spine is stabilized by the spinal extensors, abdominal engagement, and the floor. The psoas helps at the lumbar area. The upper leg, at 90 degrees, circles across, down, out, and up, completing the actions of hip adduction, extension, abduction, and flexion (this equals *circumduction*); rotation can also be added. The psoas major acts as a minimal mover at the hip joint as part of the iliopsoas muscle group, and stabilizes the spine.

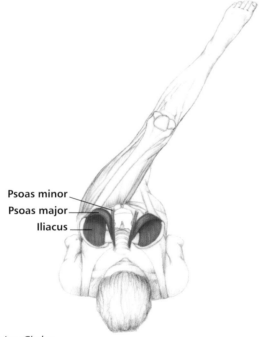

Psoas minor
Psoas major
Iliacus

*Figure 4.3: Single Leg Circles.*

4. **Rolling like a Ball**: Using a complete hip and spine flexion position, the focus of this exercise is control of the position as one rolls through the lower to mid spine on the mat. Though fun to do, some spines are just too bony or injured to be rolled on, so use caution if it is uncomfortable. The psoas works as a stabilizer, especially when balancing just behind the sit bones. The work increases on the way up from the roll to a balanced position.

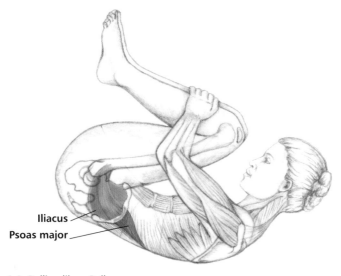

*Figure 4.4: Rolling like a Ball.*

**The next five (5 to 9) exercises are called the abdominal series. Each exercise is done 5–8 times, with even flow throughout the repetitions.**

5. **Single Leg Stretch**: The psoas will work as a weak hip and partial spine flexor, but mostly engages as it is challenged when switching from one leg to the other. This is a Level I exercise, where concentration is on the core; hip work is secondary.

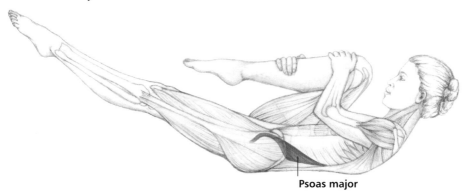

*Figure 4.5: Single Leg Stretch.*

6. **Double Leg Stretch**: This exercise is a more difficult version of the Single Leg Stretch, as both legs are extended away from the body at the same time, without use of the arms. This advanced leverage system makes the psoas work hard as a connector while the abdominals stabilize. It is a difficult exercise if the abdominals and psoas are weak.

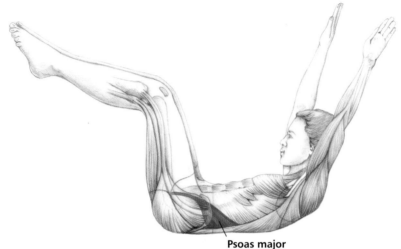

**Psoas major**

*Figure 4.6: Double Leg Stretch.*

7. **Scissors**: This is useful as a hamstring stretch, but the psoas is also engaged to a small degree in both flexion and stabilization of the hip and spine as one switches the legs. Releasing the arms forward instead of holding the leg will increase the challenge of the exercise.

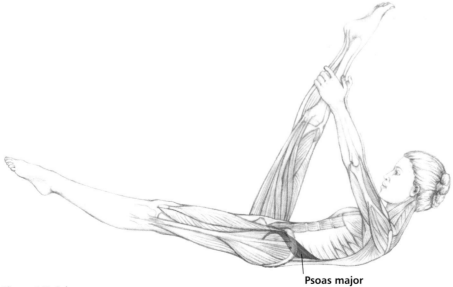

**Psoas major**

*Figure 4.7: Scissors.*

8.  **Leg Lowers**: The name describes the movement. Lowering the legs from a 90-degree position works the psoas as a stabilizer of the lumbar spine, and raising the legs back up contracts the entire iliopsoas muscle group as well as other hip flexors; working against gravity with the weight of both legs is not easy to do. To aid the lower back, bend the knees slightly as a Level I exercise, and cushion the sacral area with the hands underneath. Try to keep the spine neutral. The head and arms can be raised off the floor for added resistance.

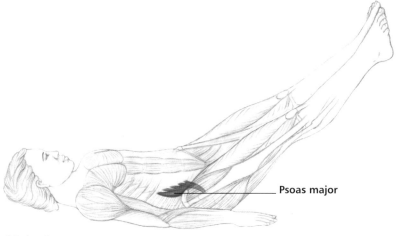

Figure 4.8: Leg Lowers.

9.  **Crisscross**: This is another psoas worker, but focuses more on the oblique abdominal muscles. The psoas acts as a stabilizer of the lower spine and as a flexor of the hip, although minimal. It will engage as a deep core muscle while the person switches from one side to the other. Do not pull on the neck with the hands; lightly touch the back of the cervical area with the elbows out, not in.

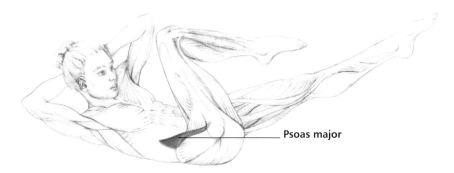

Figure 4.9: Crisscross.

10. **Spine Stretch**: In the Spine Stretch there is hip and spinal flexion, which can activate the psoas, but the spine extends against gravity in the second half of the exercise back to the vertical position. The psoas will mostly engage along with the transversospinalis muscle group to support extension of the spine on the way up from the flexed position. Sitting with the back against a wall will aid in awareness; keep the shoulders down as the spine extends.

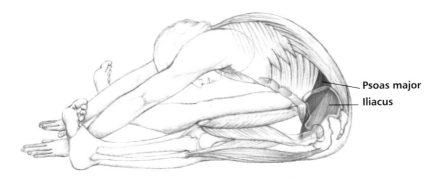

*Figure 4.10: Spine Stretch.*

Notice up to this point there has not been much stretch indicated for the psoas area and one is almost halfway through a classical Pilates mat class. This author would do the following stretch at this point.

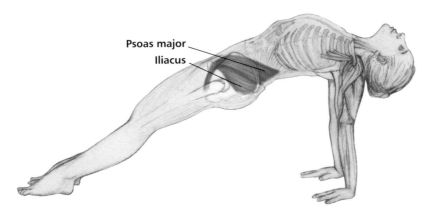

*Figure 4.11: Purvottonasana (Upward Plank Pose).*

11. **Corkscrew**: The psoas is a main worker throughout this exercise, as a stabilizer at some positions and as a mover at others. A difficult exercise for most people, it involves circling the legs together as the head, spine, and pelvis remain stable on the floor. If possible, the hips can lift at the end of a circle, engaging not only the psoas but also the deep pelvic muscles. The Kegel move (Chapter 2), which is a "squeeze" of the sit bones toward each other, can be done here if the hips are lifted at the end.

Taking the legs below 45 degrees toward the floor is not advised, and placing the hands under the sacrum will aid the lower back.

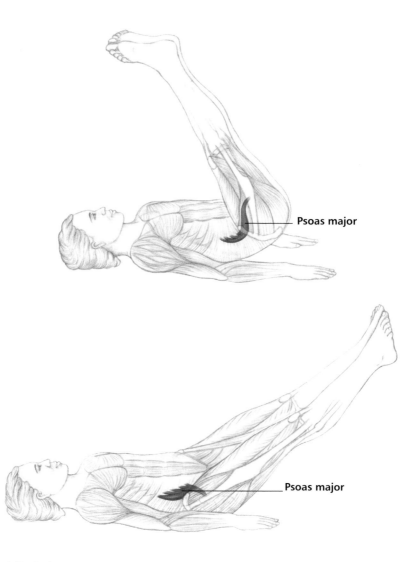

Figure 4.12: Corkscrew.

12. **The Saw**: This is similar to the spine stretch, with rotation of the spine added, where the psoas works great as a stabilizer and extensor of the lumbar spine against gravity. This is one of the most specific exercises in the Pilates system, where full attention must be paid to alignment, positioning, and core control of the entire movement; it is not about reaching the toes.

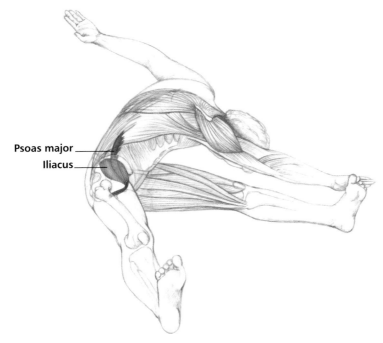

Psoas major

Iliacus

*Figure 4.13: The Saw.*

13. **Swan Prep**: Finally a psoas stretcher! The first half of this exercise emphasizes the raising of the upper extremity while the lower half remains on the floor. This will elongate the front of the hip where the psoas is located distally. The psoas also helps stabilize the lower spine.

    The second part of the exercise is to raise the lower extremity while the upper half remains on the floor, which also stretches the psoas at the front of the hip. Its supporting action at the lumbar spine is working as well.

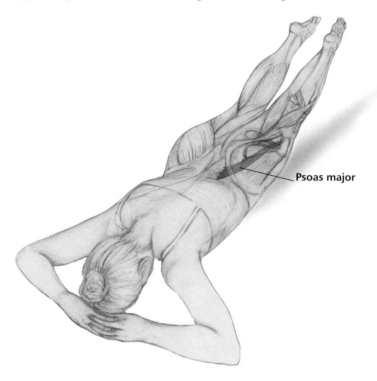

Psoas major

*Figure 4.14: Swan Prep.*

14. **Single Leg Kicks**: The psoas is slightly stretching at the front of the hip as one lies prone, propped up on the elbows, while the knees alternately bend. The core muscles, especially the abdominals and upper psoas, support the lower spine when engaged.

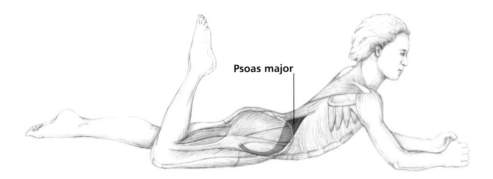

Psoas major

*Figure 4.15: Single Leg Kicks.*

15. **Child's Pose**: One of the few resting poses in the Pilates beginner mat class, it stretches the lower spine by elongation of the muscles, which includes the upper portion of the psoas. It is a released position.

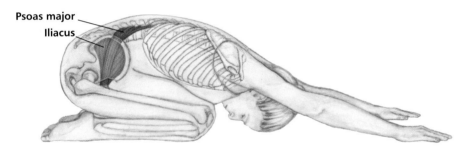

Psoas major
Iliacus

*Figure 4.16: Child's Pose.*

The psoas major helps with core *stabilization* in the following exercises. The arm position for any side-lying exercise is: Level I, head rests on outstretched bottom arm with top hand in front of chest; Level II: Lift torso and rest on bottom forearm extended in front, or as shown in Figure 4.17; Level III is shown in Figure 4.18. Five leg repetitions are usually done slowly in each exercise.

16. **Side Leg Lifts**: This exercise focuses on actions at the hip joint that the psoas is not active in, such as abduction and adduction. If the leg is externally rotated, it might incorporate the psoas to a small extent, for example as shown in the illustration below. Add circling the leg for more challenge and work.

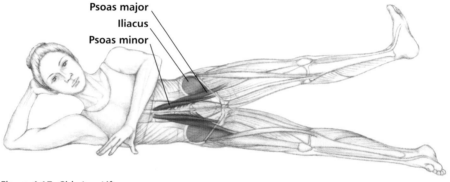

*Figure 4.17: Side Leg Lifts.*

17. **Side Leg Kicks**: This one is great for the psoas, as it works to keep the torso stable, while helping as a hip flexor. While lying on the side, the top leg kicks forward twice (hip flexion), then lengthens to the back, extending the hip. This last action stretches the psoas.

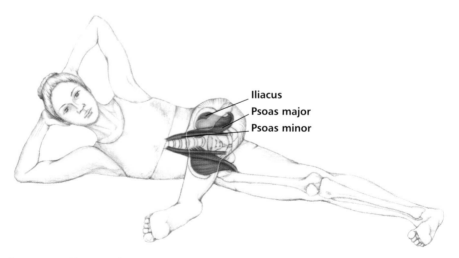

*Figure 4.18: Side Leg Kicks.*

18. **Bottom Leg Lifts**: With emphasis on the bottom leg lifting up against gravity, the hip adductors are strengthened. The psoas works more as a stabilizer during spinal extension.

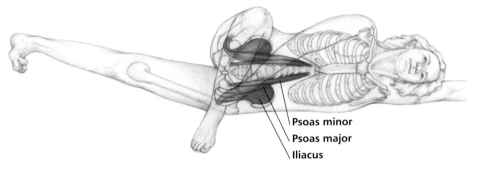

Psoas minor
Psoas major
Iliacus

*Figure 4.19: Bottom Leg Lifts.*

**Stretches:** Two stretches that could be done here are the **Half-Bridge Stretch** (for the front hip flexors such as the iliopsoas) and the **Crossed-Leg Stretch**, overleaf, (for external hip rotators, gluteals and ITB, and lower spine extensors).

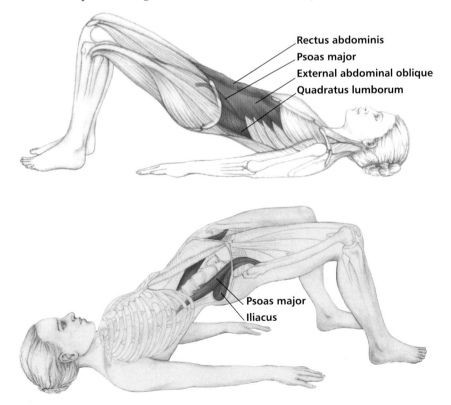

Rectus abdominis
Psoas major
External abdominal oblique
Quadratus lumborum

Psoas major
Iliacus

*Figure 4.20: Half-Bridge Stretch.*

**Crossed-Leg Stretch**: Another classic stretch is the Crossed-Leg Stretch. Lie on the back, cross the ankle of the worked leg over the other knee, and pull the bottom thigh to the chest with both hands.

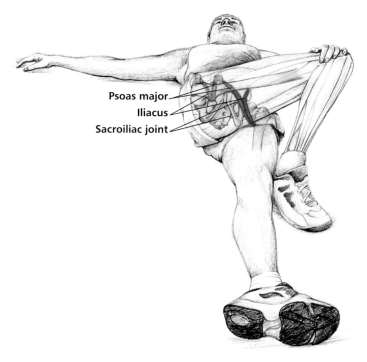

Psoas major
Iliacus
Sacroiliac joint

*Figure 4.21: Crossed-Leg Stretch.*

19. **The Half-Teaser**: Since this is a beginner mat routine list, the regular teaser is usually too difficult for novices. In Level I, do not extend both legs while lying on the floor – just one, raised to knee height; keep the other leg bent, with the foot out on the floor. Squeeze the thighs together as you roll up and down, slowly and with control. Switch legs after 3 repetitions.

This exercise is a psoas worker on the straight leg side, and stabilizer on the bent knee side.

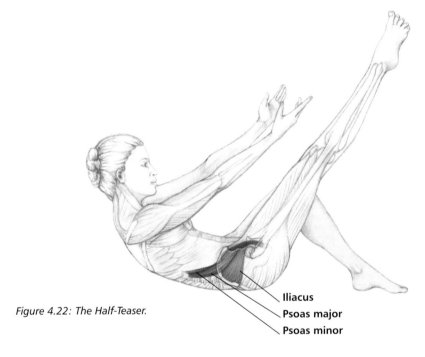

**Iliacus**
**Psoas major**
**Psoas minor**

*Figure 4.22: The Half-Teaser.*

20. **The Seal**: From a sitting position, the hips are flexed as well as the spine, with the hands holding the outside of the ankles, and the knees out to the sides, with the heels pulled in. The psoas will act as a stabilizer and core muscle throughout most of the exercise. Roll back and up through the spine three times, clapping the feet for fun at the top and bottom of the rolls. (Similar to 4. Rolling like a Ball on page 58, with outward hip rotation incorporated.)

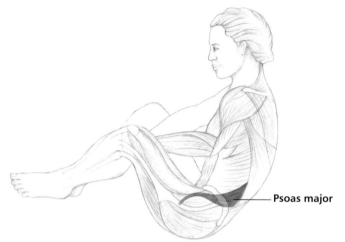

Psoas major

*Figure 4.23: The Seal.*

21. **The End:** From a standing position, roll down to the floor with the knees slightly bent, walk out on the hands, and assume a front support position. Push-ups can be added. Walk hands back to feet while engaging the core and trying not to bobble. Roll back up. The psoas helps stabilize the core throughout.

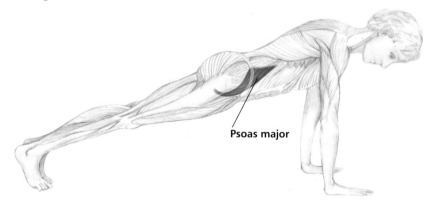

Psoas major

*Figure 4.24: The End.*

> *To reiterate, the psoas can only maintain a healthy response if other core muscles are engaged properly. Too much stress during repetitive exercise will result in imbalance and exhaustion.*

## A Note about Pilates Equipment

### Pilates Machines

The machines used in a Pilates workout can range from the Reformer only, to others such as the Wunda and High Chairs, the Trapeze, the Cadillac, the Ladder and Hump Barrels, the Pilates Stick, the Tower, and more. A fully trained Pilates personal instructor is essential as a guide while one completes a full routine. This is an intense, concentrated workout that incorporates the psoas as both a stabilizer and a mover in most exercises. Care must be taken, as in the Pilates mat class, to focus on correct muscular effort so the psoas is not overworked.

### Other Equipment

The use of Pilates rings, bands, balls, blades, ropes, rollers, ped-o-pulls, and so on are advantageous because resistance is added to challenge the workout. Original physical integrity learned in a basic mat class, and maintained, can aid anyone when equipment is added.

This author suggests that Pilates work is effective, but not in and of itself.

> *A routine of Pilates conditioning, along with yoga and walking or swimming, or even light weight training, is a great way to achieve a balance without sensitive body mechanisms being disrupted by added force or impact.*

# Part 2:
# The Psoas and Emotions

Emotions have developed over millions of years of evolution. They are the human response to nature, and in some ways protect us from harm. When we are fearful, we protect ourselves from either physical or psychological risk. If fear is extreme, it can become destructive. These feelings are harbored in the brain and linked to survival. They are part of the brain's connection with the nervous system, which links with the psoas.

# 5

# Connections –
## Somatic Memory:
## The Gut/Brain Connection

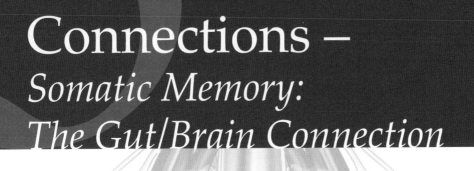

## Somatic Memory

The science of somatics is the science of the body; phrases like *somatic memory* or *somatic intelligence* mean the body's intelligence. It is now understood that people can hold embedded memories of traumatic events in the body as well as the brain. Somatic practitioners believe in the body's innate intelligence, and facilitate individual awareness of this through bodywork and other various means. Integration of the mind, body, and feelings to allow the body's non-verbal communication system to respond in a healthy way is key to healthy living. Somatic healing is about getting in touch with the "sixth sense" (intuitive response) to facilitate a breakthrough in personal health and wellness. It is about listening to a language of immediate experiences, not planned intentions or verbal messages. This is not easy to do in today's society.

How does all this include the psoas? Looking back at Part I, one can see how the deep location and connection of the psoas affects the central and peripheral nervous systems. Having a fundamental role in behavioral patterns, the memory of traumatic stress can be held in the psoas major as an organ of perception. Its involvement can cause tightness, unresponsiveness, and pain. Its release can begin a healing process.

The "fight or flight" reaction is a response of the *sympathetic* nervous system; the relaxation response for rest and recovery is through the *parasympathetic* nervous system. When one experiences overpowering stress, this healthy process may be subdued. Pent-up energy is held in the body as memory and can appear as physical symptoms. With repeated or unresolved trauma, sickness can develop.

A list of possible emotional disorders include:

- Post-traumatic stress disorder
- Acute stress disorder
- Addictions
- Syndromes (google this for an immense list)
- Depression
- Regression
- Phobias (fear of)
- Panic attacks
- Anxiety disorders
- Obsessive-compulsive disorder
- Sleep disorders
- Nightmares

These are disorders of the mind and need to be evaluated to differentiate between brain dysfunction and other sources of emotional problems. Either way, they can be held in the body. Much has been written about the psoas and its connection to our innate responses to emotions. I defer to the experts but believe that:

> *If working with a muscle can ease these problems, it could alleviate drug use for the trauma caused.*

## The Gut/Brain Connection

Suffice it to say that everything is connected to everything else. The "gut" area houses the enteric nervous system that functions, in a way, as a brain within the gut (intestines). The gut/brain connection is a phrase attracting attention as research continues to look for answers to depression, autism, and other major illnesses. The complex array of bacteria within our gastrointestinal tract and how it relates to health is still in question, but many people are beginning to believe that these bacterial organisms are capable of sending out signals, communicating with other cells and able to interpret and change environmental cues.

The enteric system receives input from the parasympathetic and sympathetic systems – all three are part of the autonomic nervous system that controls organs and muscles in the body involuntarily. There is also a *somatic* nervous system that voluntarily affects skeletal muscle. Both systems make up the peripheral nerve complex and can affect the psoas as part of the reflex of "fight or flight" in emergencies, and "rest and digest" in non-emergencies.

Impulses from the central nervous system (brain and spinal cord) can be called emotional responses, or "feelings." These may create muscle tension, which affects the psoas because of its centrality discussed before. Therefore, when the psoas is released, emotions such as fear, anxiety, and other disturbances housed in the body can surface. Once they surface and can be "let go," the entire area can become balanced and work in harmony.

## Guide to the Nervous System

The human nervous system controls, by means of neurons, the functions of all the different systems of the body. It has two parts:

1) **Central nervous system (CNS)**: encompasses the brain and the spinal cord. This system enables us to think, learn, reason, and maintain balance.

2) **Peripheral nervous system (PNS)**: located outside the brain and spinal cord, in the outer parts of the body. This system helps us to carry out voluntary and involuntary actions, and feel through the senses. The PNS comprises:

a) **Autonomic nervous system (ANS)**: responsible for regulation of internal organs and glands; it controls involuntary actions. The ANS consists of three subsystems:

   i) **Sympathetic nervous system**: activates what is commonly known as the "fight or flight" response. The psoas is considered the fight/flight muscle.

   ii) **Parasympathetic nervous system**: stimulates the "rest and digest" activities.

   iii) **Enteric nervous system**: controls the gastrointestinal system in vertebrates.

b) **Somatic nervous system (SNS)**: carries information from nerves to the CNS, and from the CNS to the muscles and sensory fibers; it is associated with voluntary muscle control.

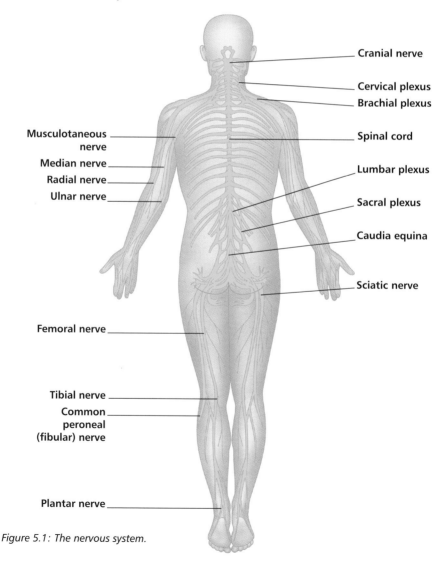

*Figure 5.1: The nervous system.*

# Nurturing the Psoas for Emotional Release

Imagine being kind to a muscle; do we ever do this? Society dictates that we work a muscle to exhaustion, whether in work or play. This is also the main principle in strength training. Let's take a different approach with the psoas, since it is probably already tired. *Freeing it* from so many chores may help to relieve emotional tension, and even trauma held deep in the core of the body.

Learning how to release it is a main focus in Chapters 2 and 6. When muscles are relaxed, they begin to affect the rest of the body and the mind. This is felt during a massage and other gentle bodywork modalities and somatics, such as Bartenieff Fundamentals. It is also experienced when one begins to fall asleep. Singling out the psoas requires openness and perception. Try the following techniques.

**Fetal Position**
1. Curl onto one side and close the eyes.
2. Envision the psoas major deep within the center of the body, supple and soft. In this position, it is really not doing any work. Instead of being in contraction, it is at rest.
3. Think of the psoas as a living, breathing organism, circulating fluid and messages in an involuntary way. It is a deep, central part of the body's universe and deserves respect and kindness.

**The Psoas "Rock"**
1. Begin a gentle rock of the pelvis, either in the fetal position or when lying on the stomach – imagine rocking a baby. Slow down to a stop when it feels right.
2. Visualize the pathways of the muscle connections – fascia, tendons, and nerve innervations – down the legs and up the spine.
3. Allow the mind to receive the subtle, calming messages of nurturing and caring from the very core. Take your time.

**The Beginner's Mind**
1. Remember how you looked and felt about things as a child: curious, unafraid, honest, free. Think of a particular situation that may help.
2. Children live in the present, from moment to moment. See and feel things as they do, not yet knowing or judging.
3. Imagine the psoas as if for the very first time – maybe it is your first time. Be open to new possibilities. This may take a while, since we tend to remain stuck in old habits. Muscles do the same thing. Use the wisdom of the body.

The *beginner's mind* approach is part of the famous stress-reduction techniques of Dr. Jon Kabat-Zinn, one of the original facilitators of mind-body medicine. Dr. Kabat-Zinn's Stress Reduction Clinic at the University of Massachusetts Medical School has become world renowned, helping millions to manage pain, tension, and disease. Among his publications are *Coming to Our Senses* and *Wherever You Go, There You Are*.

The above is all part of the practice of *mindfulness*: paying attention, not trying to control or judge things, and having patience and acceptance. It is a practice, which, if incorporated into one's daily life, can have a life-changing effect. Emotional and painful release may take place; if this is experienced, let it happen. Some people choose to do this with a qualified professional, others on their own. Either way, it can be liberating.

> *Learning to relax is a lifelong process; it is growth.*

# 6

# When the Psoas
# Strikes Back

Muscle tension is related to stress and can become detrimental. This is evident in many situations, such as upper shoulder and neck strain caused by anything from uneasy feelings, to conflict, to poor posture. This is a superficial area of the body and therefore more noticeable. Less known is the stress in deeper muscles like the psoas. Trauma can be held there for many years.

## Healing Psoas Practices

As the psoas tightens, it affects posture, placement, walking, energy, and emotions. Reaching the psoas is problematic because of its sensitivity to other structures in proximity, as well as its deep location. Therefore, it is important that *natural bodywork be done by the individual to release and relax the psoas*.

1. **CRP**: The constructive rest position can be done by anyone and, once learned, repeated as often as necessary without an instructor needed as a guide. This and other exercises can be found in Chapter 2 of Part I: "Maintaining a Healthy Psoas."

2. **Body Scan**: Lie down on the back in a quiet place, with the legs and arms outstretched. Close the eyes and begin to scan the body with the mind, sensing any tension. Start at the feet, slowly working through each joint and large muscle group; when a spot feels tense, stay there and breathe the tension away. When at the hips, pay particular attention to the deep hip crease (where the leg meets the pelvis) and really allow the stress to let go, then circle around to the sacrum and begin to release there. Continue scanning through the core and all the way up to the scalp. It really is that simple.

3. **Tension/Release**: Begin in the above position (no. 2). Starting with one leg, curl the toes and contract the muscles all the way up the thigh for a few seconds, then release. Repeat on the other leg, then the pelvic area, the torso, each arm, and the face. Finally rest, with increased awareness of release.

4. *Savasana*: This is a yoga pose (*asana*) that is done at the end of a yoga class. It is a complete rest position, usually done on the back, where the person completely lets go of not only bodily tension but also thoughts and emotions. The breath guides the person to a deep state of relaxation and opens the heart. The psoas is also released. See the end of Part III.

5. **Meditation**: Meditation is best done in a sitting position, with the hip flexor muscles relaxed and the spine lengthened to provide optimal conditions for energy flow. The above position (no. 4) can also be used if the hip flexors need to open.

Deep-seated conflicts held in the psoas can be profound; examples of this are found in the following case studies.

# Psoas Stories: Surgery, Fear, and Healing

## Ashley Ludman, Occupational Therapist, Yoga Teacher*

David entered the yoga studio for his initial evaluation session with hesitation. "I'm not sure what yoga can do for me," he stated. "The surgery didn't seem to do the trick. I am still in pain."

David is a successful general contractor in his early 50s and is very well "put together." He arrives early for his appointment, organized and ready to give this "yoga thing" a try after a friend suggested he come see me for a personalized therapeutic yoga program (his friend alleviated her back pain and frequent migraine headaches shortly after she began yoga practice earlier that year).

We started the evaluation through movement exercises. David began to share some of the background information that led him here. Prior to the moment that the "straw broke the camel's back" when he was bending over to pick up something, David's back discomfort had been growing into pain, and his orthopedic surgeon had suggested the surgical route. Months following his surgery, he was cleared to return to a restriction-free life. David was concerned that he continued to feel a nagging pain in his back that significantly limited his activities of daily living. The doctor assured David that the lumbar discectomy had taken care of the bulging disc, but David still had pain that kept him from surfing and often took his breath away if he moved into positions suddenly and without thinking it through first.

As I take David through passive range of motion, I notice a holding pattern in his hips, specifically his psoas and gluteal muscles. He continues to share other aspects of his life: work, family, demands. David has a reputation for high-quality, consistent projects; he has a full workload and many clients with large expectations. He tells me that he will often take on the demanding clients who angrily want and expect him to "jump" at unrealistic demands. "I have been dealing with this for years, I am pretty used to it by now," he comments, about dealing with the stress of such a profession.

* Ashley Ludman is owner and director of Seaside Yoga in Wilmington, North Carolina and Nosara, Costa Rica. She began working as an occupational therapist in 1996. A yoga therapist and teacher trainer, she is versed in Tantric philosophy and meditation. She can be contacted through her website: www.seasideyoga.com.

We continue to speak as I start to teach him some simple yoga postures. He notes that his muscles feel very tense, especially his hips. Lots of high and low lunges and postures to open his psoas are incorporated into his program. He learns and uses *ujjayi* breathing, and although he needs prompting of his breath throughout the yoga practice, this appears to be a good tool to settle his mind and soften out the nervous system when he becomes over-rigid and stressed.

He moves slowly and methodically, attempting all that I ask of him with a degree of fear that prevents him from fully softening into the poses. We begin to address the underlying emotion of fear, and David opens up a little further about his pain. "I guess, in a way, I am fearful of getting older and not being able to do the things that I love doing. It is challenging to be limited by this pain, especially in my job performance, because if I can't do my job, I can't care for my family the way that I need to." He continues to describe the physical aspect of the limitation. "It feels as though there is something stuck deep inside of my back, and although the doctor assures me that the disc was stabilized, it feels as though something's going to break if I push it too far."

His perception of visceral sensation was valid, and we continued to work on opening up the lumbar region, specifically the psoas, with movements such as spinal articulations. Over continuous sessions, I observed David's movement becoming more fluid. He was able to consciously create better muscle balance, incorporating deeper core integration, rather than firing off the psoas to do the primary job of articulation.

The most challenging aspect of his practice as he progressed was a full articulating sit up from supine. We began slowly, by practicing first the roll down from a seated Staff Pose (*Dandasana*), addressing his awareness of lengthening the psoas in the direction of the legs and spine during the exercise. Initially, as he progressed to the reciprocal movement (rising from supine), he would use his hands to push up from the floor. We found that if he placed a folded hand towel under his lumbar spine, he had better access to the full sit up movement while limiting the use of his hands to assist him up.

Then, it happened. One day, David came up to sitting, effortlessly articulating his spine with no pain. We both looked at each other, and he breaks down into tears. "I'm so sorry," he sobs, "I don't know where this is coming from."

"This is an emotional release," I explain. "Our bodies have a way of holding emotions deep within the cells, and oftentimes it is the emotion that actually holds the pain. Once we release what we have been holding on to, the pain leaves with it. It is good for you. Do you feel how much your body has already changed?"

"Now you are sensing that there is another layer to your strength. Beneath the external layer of what we can see, you experienced a deeper strength that also gives you the permission to surrender the clasping and holding." David walked out of the yoga studio that day with lightness in his step. His face seemed to soften a bit more. His entire body moved with a greater fluidity. It was as if he finally allowed himself to surrender.

Months later, after David had the opportunity to put his practice "on the mat" into practice "off the mat," we spoke again about letting go of fear. "Actually, I realized that beyond the emotion of fear, there was the issue of control that I had to address. I couldn't control every situation that was presented to me. It was the fear of not being in control that became the trigger for the pain. Luckily, now, I am able to sense it before it sets in, and I have tools to work with it. It is never completely gone, because it is such a deep pattern in my life, but I know now how to relate to it, and how to relate to myself."

## I Am My Own Case Study

**Jo Ann Staugaard-Jones**

I began work on this book in February of 2010, after over 30 years of intense study of modern dance, Pilates, and yoga, and an insatiable desire for sports like softball and gymnastics in the earlier days, and downhill skiing from college onward. I approached life through the physical realm – a true believer in health and physical education for all, always "on the go." Throughout my career I searched for different means of bodywork: Bartenieff Fundamentals, Alexander Technique, Feldenkrais, and Body-Mind Centering. Eventually, as a dance and kinesiology professor, I developed a strong advocacy for injury prevention through awareness. I had my own overuse injuries to contend with (knees especially) and worked to treat them naturally.

Last summer my right sacroiliac joint was acting up; it became chronic, so I sought treatment through physical therapy and chiropractic sessions. In my first visit I relayed my belief that the spot on my SI joint was directly behind scar tissue on the front of the body. After being evaluated, the therapist agreed: not only was it related, but scar tissue had begun to interfere with none other than – my *psoas major*! I have had three abdominal surgeries over my lifetime – two on my right side, and the other a cesarean.

### The Cesarean Issue

The scar tissue of the cesarean was directly related to my sacroiliac pain. *Whenever the SI joint is affected, one can surmise the psoas is also a culprit and involved in some way.* Imagine the emotional issue of the surgery, as well as the realization of the full impact of the condition over a length of time.

The post-cesarean treatment is: go home and begin to lift and hold the baby, carry the baby, and change the baby, along with all the other jobs women do. This is after having the abdominal muscles cut through to pull a fetus out. There was no physical therapy prescription, or even exercises to follow, except to "get up and move." Many years later, this travesty results in restriction of movement, poor posture, and a multitude of other complications. The compensation is a beautiful human being, thank goodness.

The causes of some injuries/conditions are stated as "incisions," which are actually injuries to the body in themselves. Lower abdominal incisions include cesareans, appendectomies, abdominal hysterectomies, inguinal hernia surgery, and abdominoplasty (tummy tuck). These not only affect the muscles, but can damage nerves as well. Laparoscopic procedures have lessened the invasion, but not entirely.

My treatment involved many hours of manipulation and pressure to the scar tissue and the psoas. The psoas at first reacted in an extremely painful way: the response of the "fight or flight" muscle was *fight*. Over time this subsided, and the therapist was able to gently soften the restrictive tissue. Only a qualified therapist should attempt this kind of work, and it is hard to tell who is. My theory is: if it is painful don't do it, unless you trust the person implicitly.

The full treatment was more "wholesome," involving stretching and strengthening of many muscles around the area, with exercises intended to develop the glutes, abdominals, psoas, hip flexors, and spinal extensors. This therapy was successful – just 25 years too late. The moral of the story is that any woman who has just given birth, even if naturally, should be in a healing situation with some kind of rehabilitation, be it physical, emotional, or spiritual.

## The Case of Groin and Testicular Pain

**Dr. Gary Mascilak, D.C., P.T., C.S.C.S.**

A 41-year-old male was presented to my office for consultation with chief complaints of right-sided testicular pain for approximately 3 to 4 months. He noted that the pain was progressive in nature and worsened with sitting, and rated the pain as a 7 out of 10 (10 being the highest amount of pain).

Lab findings were normal, with the exception of a mild elevation of liver enzymes (SGOT and SGPT). A thorough history was taken and an evaluation performed. Postural inspection revealed a moderately increased lumbar lordosis with a low right iliac crest. Leg length assessment revealed a 5/16" structural short right leg. A pelvic obliquity was also evident, with a left posterior and right anterior innominate identified. Foundational assessment revealed hyperpronation influences greater on the left than on the right. Trunk active ranges of motion were essentially within normal limits, as were the hips, with the exception of poor hip extension on the right, measuring only 10 degrees. Orthopedic maneuvers were all unremarkable, as was neurologic testing, apart from mild hypoesthesia in the L1/L2 dermatomal distribution along the inguinal and upper anterior thigh.

Palpation revealed marked tenderness and hypertonicity (extreme tension) of the right psoas major, with reproduction of the patient's chief complaint of "groin and testicular pain." (An increased lumbar lordosis can also be the result or the cause of a tight/hypertonic iliopsoas.)

Treatment consisted of moist heat application to the psoas, followed by myofascial release with simultaneous active movement of the antagonist (gluteus maximus) into hip extension, providing neurologic inhibition of the treated psoas. The goal was to free the entrapped genitofemoral nerve, which anatomically pierces the psoas major and supplies sensation to the upper anterior thigh and groin region, but in this case was causing pain due to compression. This myofascial type of release was followed by triplane stretching of the iliopsoas and activation of the inhibited gluteus maximus using a variety of exercises. The patient returned 2 days later and reported an 85–90% reduction in pain. Two follow-up treatments were scheduled to release the psoas and surrounding soft tissues, as well as for reviewing and progressing the home exercise program. Imagine his release of mental anguish along with physical pain.

## Nerve Entrapment

Many therapists have found nerve entrapment, or compression, to be the source of pain in instances that might be curable without surgery. The expression "pinched nerve" usually refers to carpal tunnel syndrome, cubital tunnel syndrome, or sciatica, but it is applicable to any pressure on a particular nerve or group of nerves.

The causes are specific to the area of concern, and can range from degenerating discs, bone spurs, arthritis, and muscle dysfunction, to injury and emotional trauma causing muscle tension, such as with the psoas. Each scenario is specific.

## Lumbar Spine Stenosis

A painful condition, lumbar spine stenosis is usually caused by degenerative arthritis or a disc disease called spondylosis. The lumbar spine is made up of many joint facets where nerves coming off the spinal cord travel through the spinal canal and openings (called foramina) on the side vertebra. When the canal or a foramen narrows or is compromised, the nerves are compacted. These nerves have an effect on the lower extremities through the path of the lumbar plexus, located behind the psoas major. Discomfort or pain is felt in the hips and legs when the nerve is compressed.

The idea is to open up the nerve passageway affected by stenosis or carpal tunnel syndrome, or any area where a nerve is inhibited. Treatments range from medications for reducing inflammation and pain, to injections, or even surgery. Depending on severity, this author would always choose physical therapy first as a less invasive alternative to medicine and surgery. As described in the above case histories, surgery was involved or suggested, when in fact the most effective treatment could have been natural bodywork, including work with the psoas. It has been proven that nerve entrapment can be opened through muscular release. I am not suggesting that this is the case with spinal stenosis, but prevention through diet and bodywork and early detection can certainly reduce the number of cases and surgeries.

The nervous system is extremely complex. Try to follow the pathway of just one component: the genitofemoral nerve. This nerve

- is part of the upper region of the lumbar plexus;
- originates from L1 and L2 nerve roots;
- emerges on the anterior surface of the psoas major muscle;
- divides into a femoral and genital branch;
- supplies the skin anterior to the upper part of the femoral triangle;
- in males, travels through the inguinal canal, supplying the cremaster muscle (covering the testis) and scrotal skin;
- in females, ends in the skin of the mons pubis (anterior portion of the vulva) and the labia majora (inner vagina lips).

> *The psoas even becomes a factor in sexual arousal.*
> *What a great reason to maintain its health!*

There are many other psoas stories – positive proof that working with the release of the psoas can achieve dramatic results. Some of the best psoas work is done by Liz Koch, international educator and somatic practitioner. Her website is www .coreawareness.com. As she explains:

> *"The psoas is no ordinary muscle but a profound segue into the rich, inner and outer world of awareness and consciousness."*

We are now ready to begin the journey into the spiritual aspect of human (and psoas) potential, Part III.

# Part 3: The Psoas and Spirituality – "Energetic" Anatomy

It is the author's intent that this third part open people up to the possibilities of energy work in correlation with physical exercise and anatomy. Examining the body's center of power, movement, and equilibrium includes the psoas major muscle as an integral force. The spiritual chakra system that is tapped in focused energy work is also located here, specifically the lower three chakras. If the psoas is used correctly, it will not inhibit the spiritual process, but help to complete it. This theory will be explored throughout this part.

# What Do We Know?

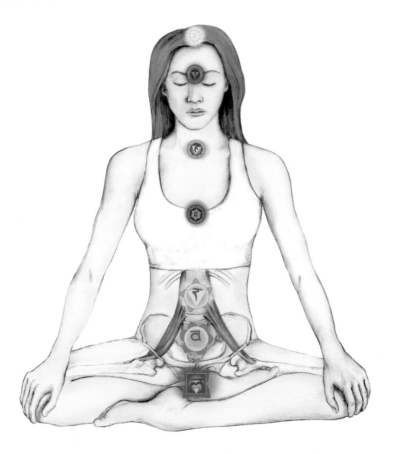

## Science and Spirituality

It has finally been scientifically proven that there are two unique levels of physical reality: the one we are familiar with (using the five senses) and a second one termed *psychoenergetic* science. This is a level of physical reality that can be significantly influenced by human intention. Stanford University professor and physicist William A. Tiller, PhD, is associated with this finding, namely that the expansion of traditional science to include human consciousness and human intention as capable of significantly affecting both the properties of materials (non-living and living) and what we call physical reality is possible. Einstein and quantum physics opened the door to this concept of creativity and transformation at the beginning of the twentieth century.

Are we on the cusp of a new scientific worldview that encompasses the growth of consciousness? We know we have many unrealized capabilities. Wouldn't it be wonderful to be able to affect reality toward a common good, using a conscious power? It seems that up until now this has only been addressed spiritually, mainly through yoga/meditation, metaphysical practices, and energy healing.

The link between science and spirituality is definitely overdue and ripe for investigation. What does this have to do with the "almighty psoas?" Remembering the psoas connection from Parts I and II – the physical and the emotional – a definite relationship between brain chemistry and physical/emotional health has been proven. Knowing that the psoas major muscle is located within the solar plexus, how can this muscle not also be related to the spiritual chakras and their effect on the well-being and intent of the person? This is not as a transmitter of energy, however, but more as an "enabler" when it is in a non-contracted (free) state. The link between the health of the psoas and the chakra system will be presented with yoga *asanas* (postures) to enhance the process.

## The Chakra System: The Cosmic Self

The *cakras* (original spelling) come from an ancient tradition, the word appearing in India a few thousand years ago at the time of an invasion by Indo-European peoples (Aryans). This became known as the *Vedic* period, when a cultural mixing took place throughout India over the following centuries. The chakra was symbolically shown as a ring of light, with a historical meaning "to bring in a new age." Chakras are mentioned in the Vedas, the ancient Hindu text of knowledge.

Though a mystery from the past, we know the Sanskrit word *chakra* itself means "wheel," as in the wheel of time, believed also to be a metaphor for the sun, therefore representing celestial balance. Yogic literature mentions the chakras as psychic centers of consciousness as early as 200 B.C. in Patanjali's Yoga Sutras. The chakras as energy centers became an integral part of Yoga philosophy through the Tantric tradition in the seventh century A.D., where integration of the many forces of the universe was emphasized. Yoga began to incorporate the whole being.

There are seven basic chakras (other minor ones in the extremities) that work together as a complete system, sometimes called the *inner organs of the esoteric (obscure) body*, and found along the spine. They intersect with the nadis (spinal energy channels) as well as the endocrine system and nerve plexi. One could call the chakras *psychoenergetic* centers; they link to the natural elements of earth, water, fire, air, and ether, and their qualities help define human purpose. They are believed to receive, digest, distribute, and transmit life energy, and hence known as the seven roots of awakening. The psoas major intertwines the bottom three chakras.

The seven primary chakras are listed here, including the Sanskrit word for each; the sacred, ancient language of Sanskrit is revered as being designed for enlightenment, as are the chakras. The meaning and effects of the chakra system go way beyond what is indicated in this book, where energy flow and auric fields are best described by other experts such as Barbara Brennan and Cyndi Dale.

**1. Root Chakra – *Muladhara***
foundation; primal needs; grounding; connected; security
color: red; planet: Saturn; element: earth; sense: smell
location: above the anus, base of the spine, pelvic floor
governs feet, legs, large intestine
animal: elephant; root sound: *lam*
*Kundalini Shakti coils here, power of the divine feminine*

**2. Sacral Chakra – *Svadhisthana***
womb; emotional/sex flow; sweetness; pleasure; creativity
color: orange; planet: Pluto/Moon; element: water; sense: taste
location: front face of lower spine, pelvis, sacrum, ovaries, testes
governs fertility, lower back and hips, bladder, kidneys
animal: crocodile; root sound: *vam*
*expansion of one's own individuality*

**3. Solar Plexus Chakra – *Manipura***
gut feelings, breath; warrior (courage); brilliant jewel; personal power
color: yellow; planet: Sun/Mars; element: fire; sense: sight
location: solar plexus, union of diaphragm, psoas, organs,
centered around the navel
governs digestion, metabolism, emotions, universality of life
animal: ram; root sound: *ram*
*influences the immune, nervous, and muscular systems*

**4. Heart Chakra – *Anahata***
divine acceptance; love; relationships; passion; joy of life
color: green/pink; planet: Venus; element: air; sense: skin
location: upper chest, heart, lungs, thymus gland
governs upper back, psychic ability, some emotions, openness to life
animal: antelope; root sound: *yam*
*engulfs the rhythm of the universe*

**PART 3**

### 5. Throat Chakra – *Vishuddha*
communication; self-expression; harmony; vibration; grace; dreams
color: sky blue; planet: Mercury/Jupiter; element: ether; sense: hearing
location: throat, neck, thyroid, ears, mouth
governs sound, the power of the voice, assimilation
animal: white elephant; root sound: *ham*
*communicates inner truth to the world, ascends physical to spiritual*

### 6. Brow Chakra – *Ajna*
third eye; intuition; concentration; conscience; devotion; neutrality
color: indigo/purple; planet: Neptune; element: light; sense: the mind
location: center of head between and above eyebrows, pituitary gland
governs creativity, imagination, understanding, rational dreaming
animal: black antelope; root sound: *om*
*provides opportunity to see everything as sacred*

### 7. Crown Chakra – *Sahasrara*
pure consciousness; spirituality; true wisdom; integration; bliss
color: white, also violet/gold; planet: Uranus/Ketu; beyond elements
location:  top of the head, pineal gland, cerebral cortex
governs all functions of the body and mind, other chakras
symbol: thousand-petaled lotus (void)
*Kundalini energy (Shakti) unites with male energy, (Shiva) to transcend into*
*the essence of all*

This text will focus on the chakra relationship to the physical body, specifically the lower spine. As chakras of the subtle body are vitalized, so are the physical energies, especially those of the lower torso where the psoas lies.

One of the goals of a yoga practice is to free prana, defined as energy, the breath, the life force. *Kundalini* is this untapped prana found at the base of the spine, sometimes represented as a coiled snake. The root chakra is located here, as a grounding force that connects one to the earth energies. The psoas muscle interconnects this area, as well as the second and third chakras – the Sacral Chakra and Solar Plexus Chakra.

The seven basic chakras, or energy centers, are said to exist within the "subtle body" (non-physical), which overlies the physical body. Modern science has found that these areas correspond closely to the seven main nerve ganglia coming from the spinal column. The nerve centers are mentioned in Parts 1 and 2, and are directly related to the psoas through the lumbar plexus, as described at the end of Chapter 6.

When working with the chakras, one of the most important things to remember is that the system is a *whole* system, therefore they must be balanced, in harmony with one another. The same is true of the physical body.

# The Psoas and
# Chakra 1:
# "Kinesthetic Balance"

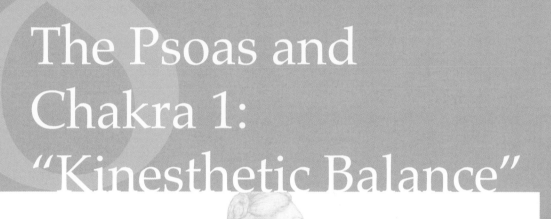

It has already been stated that the psoas interconnects the root chakra, as it is located along the base of the spine and the pelvic floor. The skeletal structure of the pelvic floor comprises the coccyx (tail bone), the pubis (pubic bone), and the ischial tuberosities (sit bones). These points intersected make up a square, and the symbol for the root chakra is also a square, or four-leafed lotus flower. *"There are no coincidences."*

There is a pose named after this chakra, Pose of the Root Lock, or *Mulabandhasana* (*mula* = root, foundation; *bandha* = binding; *asana* = posture). Usually a Level II pose, it is a combination of *Baddha Konasana* (see the following chapter on the second chakra) and the Easy Pose below. This posture is considered an advanced meditation position, as it is held for a long time while practicing *pranayama* (breathing techniques). *Bandhas* are classic efforts of binding found in most yoga, meditation, and *kriya* (action) practices, best learned from a qualified yoga master. Difficult to explain, they bring one through a reconfigured energy flow in order to achieve union between inner and outer universal forces. There is so much more to this practice than explained here, but suffice it to say the psoas major, as a unifying, central body force, is involved in some way.

## Yoga Poses and Chakra 1

The psoas can affect this area as a receptor and a preceptor (teacher). It can be activated for this first chakra through sitting yoga *asanas*, as well as in any pose involving the feet and legs. When the psoas and quadratus lumborum, as well as the pelvic floor muscles are engaged, they stabilize the lumbar and sacral areas and position the pelvis toward and into the ground. This is important in all the following poses.

Yoga positions are usually held for three full breaths or longer, depending on the instruction. A flowing sequence (*vinyasas* such as Sun Salutation) might also be included.

One must keep in mind that most yoga postures were created a few thousand years ago and are constantly evolving. They prepare the body for the spiritual work of meditation and refine the nervous system, unlocking chakra energy. There are emotional issues of survival, security, and family that are addressed in this first chakra, as well as conditions such as depression, sciatica, varicose veins, and rectal problems. The root chakra is believed to store feelings such as loyalty, superstitions, and instincts.

**Imagine the possibilities of opening this energy system to healing, by establishing a healthy sense of grounding, eliminating "garbage," and taking care of the body in a natural, caring way!** Living in the body instead of always in the brain would do much for the industrialized and technological society many of us live in.

Sitting postures affect the root chakra by harnessing the essence of the earth itself. In this way the following *asanas* take the journey from the physical to the spiritual. The psoas is active as a spine stabilizer and mostly released at the hip. Its misuse will inhibit the flow of energy.

## Sitting Postures

I. Easy Pose, *Sukhasana*, Level I
(*sukha* in Sanskrit translates as gentle, happy, or agreeable)

**Technique**: This is a still, sitting pose that optimizes the vertical length of the spine, and one that is ideal for meditation and the start of any yoga class. Sit with a straight spine, shoulders relaxed back and down, and crossed legs.

**Limitations**: Although many people feel comfortable in this position, some may find it restrictive through the knees or hips. If this is the case, the front leg can be placed out to the side, or one can sit higher on blankets or a block to allow the legs to relax with gravity's assistance. Having the hips above the knees reduces fatigue and increases flow of energy and breath. A wall can also be used to help straighten the spine, or a chair if sitting on the floor is not possible.

II. Seer Pose, *Siddhasana*, Level I
(*siddha* translates as perfected beings)

**Technique**: This is similar to Easy Pose, with the feet tucked under the legs so that the toes are not seen. The spine is straight with the shoulders pulled back and down. The breath becomes the focus of any sitting meditation pose.

**Variation**: Add a forward bend to the posture, reaching the arms forward while keeping the sit bones on the floor.

**Limitations**: Same as Easy Pose above. If doing the variation, spinal flexion is contraindicated for those with vertebral disc problems.

III. Lotus Pose, *Padmasana*, Level II
(*padma* = lotus, the symbol of creation)

**Technique**: Sitting in Easy Pose (*Sukhasana*), the feet are then placed on top of the thighs while maintaining the lift of the body. This is a powerful posture.

**Limitations**: If there are ankle, knee, or hip problems, keep working in *Sukhasana* so there is not as much strain. Eventually, as the body gets stronger, looser, and more balanced, the Lotus Pose might be achieved, trying one leg for a while, then both; or using support under the knee or hip. One must listen to the body and may not be able to achieve full Lotus, which is fine. Accepting limitations and honoring the body for what it can do is part of the yogic process.

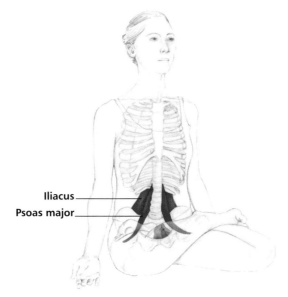

*Figure 8.1: Lotus Pose, Padmasana, Level II.*

*Kundalini* (Sanskrit for "coiled") was mentioned earlier; there are many Kundalini yoga exercises that can deeply affect the lower chakras, of which the psoas is a part. As an example, one would do Easy Pose, and begin to hyperextend the spine forward on the inhalation, and flex it backward on the exhalation, increasing the pace and doing this for a few minutes. This movement with the breath invigorates the core and the chakras, opening to increased awareness. The use of *Breath of Fire* (a sort of panting through the nose, with the navel center involved) is also used in Kundalini exercises.

Try twisting to the left on an inhalation and to the right on the exhalation with the hands on the shoulders, elbows out, increasing speed. The spine and chakras release and open. This is very powerful, as it can take one to a higher state of consciousness.

*Kundalini awakening is best served through a master teacher.*

IV. Staff Pose, *Dandasana*, Level I
(*danda* = stick or staff)

**Technique**: Sit on the floor with legs straight out in front, feet flexed, and the spine straight. Place the heels of the hands onto the floor at the sides of the hips. This is harder than it looks. The focus is alignment and breath, with energy flow in two directions: from the sit bones up the spine through and out of the crown chakra, and from the sit bones through the legs and out through the feet to engage the muscles. Working the feet will also stimulate this chakra.

**Limitations**: If one has trouble sitting up with legs straight, do not compromise the position by bending the spine – just bend the knees or place a blanket underneath them. This is usually due to tight hamstrings.

V. Half Sitting Twist, *Ardha Matsyendrasana*, Level I
(*ardha* = half; *matsyendra* = lord of the fishes)

This is a basic seated twisting posture that invigorates the root chakra as well as the rest of the spine, like all twists do. There are many muscles that are activated in the legs, spine, and arms (depending on the arm position). It is thought to have been developed by and named after a renowned yoga teacher, Sage Matsyendra.

**Technique**: Sit with one leg tucked under, and the other leg crossed over, foot flat on the floor. Extend the spine and hold the top knee with the opposite hand, or place the opposite elbow against it for more twist. Use the back arm behind the tailbone, with the hand on the floor for support. The psoas will help support the lumbar spine; it is the thoracic and cervical areas of the spine that will be able to twist (rotate) more effectively, as the lower spine is limited in rotation and should not be forced. (See figure 8.2.)

This author has seen lower back injuries directly related to yoga and believes forced twisting of the lumbar spine is one of the causes. In fact, anything forced is not the yogic way. Find a certified instructor that understands this, and kinesiology, the science of motion.

**Limitations**: The hips may actually limit the pose, as many people cannot sit on both sit bones in this position, because of tightness or even simple anatomical differences. Try extending the bottom leg and/or putting the top foot inside the lower leg instead of outside. There is also much "countermovement" going on, as one part rotates opposite to another. Flexibility helps here, so practice the pose often, and activate the root chakra by grounding both hips down into the floor and extending up through the spine.

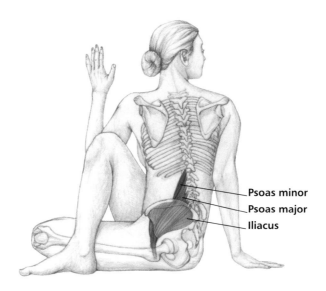

Figure 8.2: Half Sitting Twist, Ardha Matsyendrasana, Level I.

VI. Cow-Faced Pose, *Gomukhasana*, Level II
(*go* = cow; *mukha* = face)

**Technique**: Sit with the knees bent, one knee over the other, feet out to the sides on their outside edges. The spine elongates, and arm variations are possible. This is a very good grounding position.

**Limitations**: This one is a compromising position for the knees. If any stress is felt, tissue can be negatively affected. Sitting in any easier position with "cow arms" can be a variation.

VII. Boat Pose, *Navasana*, Level II
(*nava* = boat; *asana* = posture)

**Technique**: From a sitting position, raise the knees into the chest and balance just behind the sit bones. Extend one leg and then the other to a 45-degree position, if possible. The core must be engaged for correct balance and support. The arms can be extended forward for more challenge. Do not collapse the lower back – the psoas major is working here as well as at the hip joint.

**Limitations**: If the psoas muscle is weak, this position will be hard to hold and stabilize. Place the hands on the floor for balance as the thighs are brought anteriorly toward the chest with the knees bent, to ease the pose. Cushion the tailbone with a thicker support for less pressure on the lower back. If held correctly, this posture will not compress the lumbar spine, but extend it.

## Standing Postures

VIII. Mountain Pose, *Tadasana*, Level I
(*tada* = mountain)

**Technique**: This is the standing foundational pose of yoga, where the feet are rooted into the ground, parallel, for a stable base of support as the body extends upward. Harmony, centeredness, and balance are the focus. The psoas works to position the spine, pelvis, and legs in correct alignment with each other. Feet are placed either together or hip width apart, depending on the tradition.

**Limitations**: None.

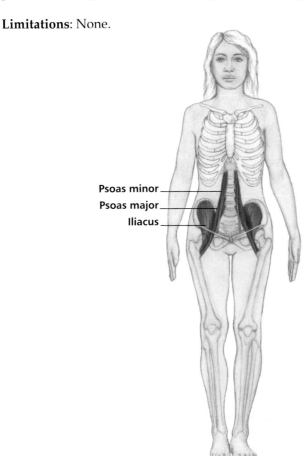

Psoas minor
Psoas major
Iliacus

*Figure 8.3: Mountain Pose, Tadasana, Level I.*

IX. Warrior I and II, *Virabhadrasana*, Level I
(*virabhadra* = brave warrior)

In hip flexion of the front leg, the psoas is contracted as part of the iliopsoas muscle group, as it helps lengthen the lower spine. The psoas is stretched at the hip joint in the back leg.

**Technique for Warrior I**: From Mountain Pose, take a large step back with one leg, keeping the hips forward. Turn the back foot in, 45 to 60 degrees. Keeping the outer edge of the back foot securely into the ground, bend the front knee directly over the front ankle, with slight outward rotation at the hip. There should be a strong, balanced stance, with equal weight on both legs. Arm positions can vary from hands on hips, to "cactus" arms, to extending above. Repeat on the other side.

**Technique for Warrior II**: Keeping the leg position of Warrior I, open the hips and arms to the side. The back toes may move out more to aid the open hips. The gaze is directly over the front hand, strong and proud.

**Limitations**: Try not to create tension in the pose, as this will limit breath and stretching. Arms above the head in Warrior I is not recommended for those with untreated high blood pressure.

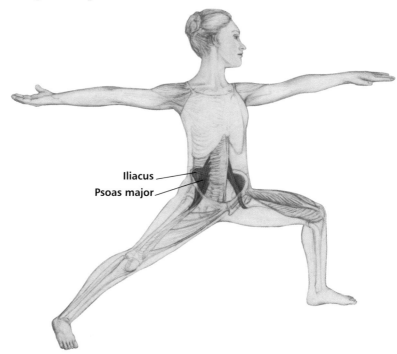

Iliacus
Psoas major

*Figure 8.4: Warrior II, Virabhadrasana, Level I.*

X. Tree Pose, *Vrksasana*, Level II
(*vrksa* = tree)

**Technique**: Stand on one leg, toes facing straight ahead, and place the other foot against the inner thigh or calf, rotating the hip outward. Extend the body upward, while the tail bone drops down. Hands can be in prayer position or high above the head. The supported leg is strengthened, while the other leg is stretched. The psoas works in both leg positions as the pelvis remains centered.

*Any one-leg balance is ideal for the root chakra, as the foot and leg are grounded into the floor and the core is engaged strongly.*

**Limitations**: Tight hips will cause the top foot to be lowered to the calf or floor (never against the knee), which is fine as long as external rotation of the hip is maintained. If one has trouble with dizziness, vertigo, or balance, hold on to a wall or support. Keep the eyes open and focused for better balance.

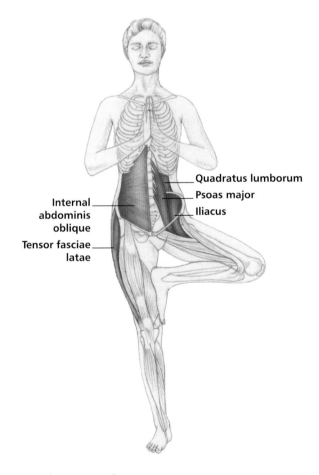

Quadratus lumborum
Psoas major
Iliacus
Internal abdominis oblique
Tensor fasciae latae

*Figure 8.5: Tree Pose, Vrksasana, Level II.*

The above ten poses are meant as a guide to help increase strength, flexibility, circulation, and activation of this area, and are by no means a complete list. End the session with a **Child's Pose** for a nice stretch.

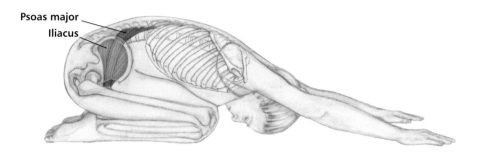

*Figure 8.6: Child's Pose, Balasana, Level I.*

## Pointers for Chakra 1

1. Try marching, stomping, and running, or even walking will do. The psoas will help to balance the transfer of weight.

2. Feel the self grounded through the earth and connect with it.

3. Eat root vegetables such as garlic, onion, carrots, beets, potatoes, radishes, and horseradish.

4. Take care of the immune system.

5. Stimulate the feet by massage.

6. Allow the "survival" instinct to take root and flourish.

7. Release the psoas and give it a rest.

## Bonus Poses

Horse Pose, *Ashvasana*, Level I/II/III
(*ashva* = horse)
(Level I: Lying on back    Level II: Standing    Level III: One-leg stance)

There are many different descriptions of this pose – the best way to understand it is to position the legs the way one would sit on a horse, either lying down or standing. The legs are strengthened as the thighs are flexed and abducted; the knees are bent over the toes.

Level III is known as *Vatayanasana*, the Flying Horse Pose, and is contraindicated for women, and for people with knee injuries. Men use it as a genital conditioner, as it is said to "moisturize" the genital nerve complex; therefore, the Level III position becomes a suggested posture for the next chakra discussed.

Most sources agree that any of the three levels circulates the blood, boosts the immune system, and strengthens the anus area.

Kundalini Crow Pose, *Bakasana*, Level I/II
Level I: Hands on floor
Level II: Prayer position

This pose is ideal for the root chakra, as gravity pulls the tailbone down and stretches the lower back. It stimulates the elimination system, relaxes the psoas, connects the mind/body to the earth, and can provide feelings of security. It increases flexibility in the hips and groin area; if there is a knee or ankle injury, care should be taken not to squat too low. (One can also do a Chair Pose, *Utkatasana*, instead to ease stress on the knees and ankles.)

Stand upright with the feet shoulder width apart, then bend the knees and squat to the floor, with the feet either parallel or turned out, knees follow the line of the foot. Heels pressed down is ideal, but only possible if the Achilles tendon is long enough. If not, a support can be placed under the heels. The hands can remain on the floor for balance (Level I) or taken to prayer position (Level II). Breath of Fire can be added.

PART 3

Chapter 8 – The Psoas and Chakra 1: "Kinesthetic Balance"

## Review: Fact or Fiction?

### Yoga is a system of exercises.

Fact – the physical asanas (postures) are arrangements of exercises that lead to health of the body, mind, and spirit.

### Yoga is a religion.

Fiction – yoga is not an organization based on beliefs, but becomes a way of life rooted in universality. The word yoga can be interpreted as "union."

### Yoga postures have different levels.

Fact – most of us like to think we can do anything, but, depending on one's body, many postures may be difficult. The levels indicated in this text can act as a guide, but it is up to the individual to determine his or her own capability, by simply being aware.

### The chakras are valid.

Fact – this author's research indicates the connection between ancient beliefs regarding energy centers of consciousness, and the more recent scientifically proven link between matter and energy.

### Muscles and energy centers are connected.

Fact – location can determine this connection, as well as deliberate breath work (through muscles such as the diaphragm and abdominals). The relaxation of muscles can also affect energy in a positive way, as with the psoas.

## Benefits of Postures

- sitting poses create openness, extension, and space in the spine, as well as calm, secure feelings of connection.
- standing poses stimulate body systems, teach correct alignment, and improve circulation, strength, and joint mobility.
- twists activate organs and create flexibility in the neck, shoulders, and lower back, as well as improving digestion and eliminating toxins.
- inversions improve concentration, activate glands, strengthen the nervous system, and invigorate the entire body.
- backbends open the chest and heart, create energy and courage, combat depression, and promote flexibility of the spine and shoulders.
- balancing poses develop muscle tone, coordination, and concentration, along with strength and flexibility.
- prone and supine poses provide the many benefits of strength, stretch, mobility, and restfulness, depending on the posture.

# 9

# The Psoas and
# Chakra 2:
# "Flow like Water"

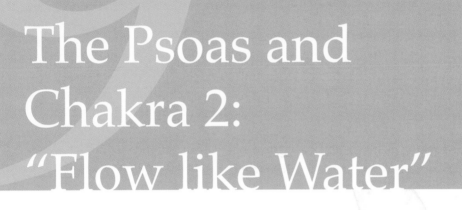

This chakra deals with sexual and other organs in the pubic region. Awareness and release of the psoas in this area can help the bladder, as well as aid in menstrual problems and pregnancy because of its proximity. Male organs can also be affected, as the genitofemoral nerve arises from the lumbar plexus, the group of nerves that originate in the lower area of the spine. This nerve innervates the upper inner thigh and the genital regions. The nerve can be affected by surgical techniques, trauma, or diseases that have an effect on the nervous system. Nerve entrapment can happen anywhere in the body, and this area is especially prone to inhibition. A neurologist would determine the extent and cause.

In this particular area, there is also the ilioinguinal nerve that emerges from the lateral border of the psoas major. It supplies branches to the transversus abdominis and internal oblique muscles, as well as to the pubic symphysis, femoral triangle, female labia, and root of the penis and scrotum in the male. Therefore, *the psoas is directly related to orgasm!* More details on this are found at the end of Chapter 6.

## Yoga Poses and Chakra 2

The following poses will stimulate the psoas and surrounding tissue of this very sacred, sacral area. Do not muscularly hold the psoas as these are performed, since tension will reduce flow.

The *bandha* here is the *uddhiyana*. Whereas the root *bandha* (*mulha bandha*) engages a grounded quality, *uddhiyana* means "upward flying," establishing lightness to the body. Being aware of the psoas, its length and positioning on both sides of the central body, can aid in this feeling.

## Sitting Postures

I. Cobbler Pose, ***Baddha Konasana***, Level I
(*baddha* = bound; *kona* = angle)

**Technique**: Sit in a strong, still position (*Sukhasana*), then open the legs and bend the knees out to the sides. Bring the soles of the feet together and draw the heels in toward the pubis. Hold the ankles. Bending forward may increase stimulation to the second chakra and the psoas.

**Limitations**: Tight hips will cause the knees to be high or the spine to bend. Sit up on blankets or a block to allow the thighs to relax, or place support under the knees. (If one knee is higher, that side has the tighter hip.) Bending forward is not suggested for those with lumbar disc problems.

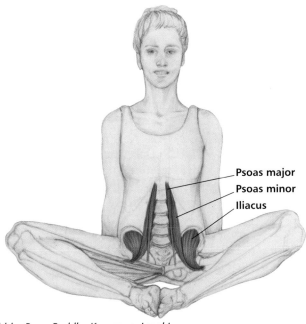

Psoas major
Psoas minor
Iliacus

*Figure 9.1: Cobbler Pose, Baddha Konasana, Level I.*

II. Hero Pose**, *Virasana*, to Reclined Hero Pose, *Supta Virasana*, Level II**
(*vira* = hero, chief)

**Technique**: Begin kneeling, with the sit bones on the floor while the feet are directly outside the hips. Lean back to place the elbows and forearms on the floor. (One can also lie on a bolster or blanket.) If there is no strain, lower the torso to the floor. This position stretches the lower psoas.

**Limitations**: If sitting upright is uncomfortable, a block or blanket may be used under the sit bones or between the thighs and calves, as raising the hips will accommodate the knees to an easier bend. Reclining the torso makes it especially difficult on the knees, as they are placed at a very deep angle. This is not suggested for anyone with knee issues.

III. Sitting Spinal Twist**, *Bharadvajasana*, Level I**
(*bharadvaja* = name of ancient sage)

This twist of course affects all chakras, but especially opens and stimulates the sacral area as the twist is taken further while the sit bones remain on the floor. Both sides of the psoas are activated differently – almost counter-stretched.

**Technique**: Sit and bend both legs to one side, with knees pointing forward. Extend and twist the spine to the opposite side of the legs. Hands are placed on the front knee and behind the hip on the floor for support.

**Limitations**: If sitting is uncomfortable, place a blanket under the hip to ease the posture.

IV. Seated Angle Pose, ***Upavista Konasana***, Level II/III
(*upavista* = seated; *kona* = angle)

**Technique for Level II**: Begin in Staff Pose, then spread the legs apart in a straddle position with knees straight and facing up. Keeping the spine erect will aid gynecological problems; this can be practiced during pregnancy or menstruation, against a wall.

**Technique for Level III**: One can extend the spine forward, holding the toes. The deep piriformis muscle (a culprit in sciatica) will work here, as well as the hip adductors stretching intensely. The psoas is stretched in spine extension, but released in hip flexion since there is no resistance to gravity. *Do not do this variation while pregnant.*

**Limitations**: Tight hamstrings, spinal extensors (of which part of the psoas is one), or hip adductors (muscles of the inside thigh) will make it harder to do this pose. Sit up on a blanket for support, or bend the knees slightly. Do not flex the spine, but elongate.

## Standing Postures

V. Forward Bends
Standing Forward Bend, ***Uttanasana***, Level I
Sitting Forward Bend, ***Paschimottanasana***, Level II
(*uttan* = extension, intense stretch; *pascha* = behind, after, west)

**Technique for Standing Forward Bend**: From Mountain Pose, flex the spine forward and reach for the floor, with the knees slightly bent and head extended in line with the spine. Go into and out of the pose slowly. (Always try to come out of a pose in the reverse way of going into it: "rewind" slowly.) The posture can be deepened with the belly and chest against the thighs, breathing to stimulate organs of this chakra area; try to relax the psoas.

**Limitation**: If there is lumbar disc injury, it is best to keep the lower spine flat instead of rounded so as not to compress the area. This is true of any forward bend variety. The posture will not be as deep as shown in the figure.

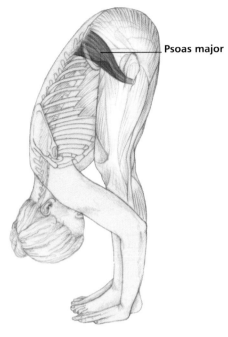

*Figure 9.2: Standing Forward Bend, Uttanasana, Level I.*

**Technique for Sitting Forward Bend**: Sit in Staff Pose and reach the hands toward the toes with an extended, not bent, spine; flex from the hips.

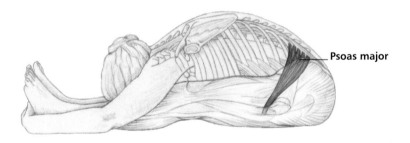

*Figure 9.3: Sitting Forward Bend, Paschimottanasana, Level II.*

**Limitations**: Tight spinal extensors (the posterior muscles that work the spine) or hamstrings will limit these poses. Bending the knees will loosen the hamstring attachment at the knees, while relaxed hip flexion will release the lower psoas. One can also sit on a higher support in the Sitting Forward Bend. An easier way to accomplish the pose is to use one leg at a time, as in *Janu Sirsasana* (Head to Knee Pose). Lower back problems can be aggravated in a full spinal flexion position, so do not overdo or overstretch. Listen to the body. This asana is best done in an extended spine position; rounding of the back can be added, as shown in figure 9.3.

VI. Standing Straddle, *Prasarita Padottanasana*, Level I/II
(*prasarita* = spread out; *pada* = foot; *uttan* = extension)

**Technique for Level I**: Begin in a wide straddle stance with hands on the hips, feet forward. Bend the spine forward, maintaining a flat back. Place the hands on the floor. Allow the sacral area to spread. This pose is a great beginning inversion, which aids blood flow to the brain. Try to release the psoas; gravity will help.

**Technique for Level II**: A deeper stretch is obtained by lowering the back and placing the elbows or top of the head on the floor.

**Limitations**: Tight hamstrings or sacral/lumbar area will limit the stretch of this pose – bend the knees to aid the lower back and release the hamstrings.

VII. Triangle, *Trikonasana*, Level I/II
(*trikona* = three angle)

This is a classic and popular yoga pose – the hips are open, allowing the psoas major to stretch, strengthen, and "breathe."

**Technique**: Begin in Mountain Pose, then separate the legs into a straddle. The foot positions are the same as for Warrior II – the front foot straight forward and the back foot turned approximately 60 degrees. The arms are out, and both legs are straight without locking the knees. Lean the torso forward toward the front hand as the back hip pushes backward. Tilt the torso, placing the front hand on the inside of the front leg; the back arm lifts up to the ceiling. The body remains in one plane.

**Limitations**: So many muscles come into play in this pose; therefore, tightness in any of them can affect the posture. Hyperextension of the knees is common, so "micro-bending" the front knee will help. (Micro-bending is a term used in yoga, meaning a tiny bend or a softening behind the knee joint.) If the shoulder is tight, place the top hand on the sacrum. The work in this pose lies in opening the hips and lengthening the spine, breathing deeply. As practice continues, amazing results can be achieved.

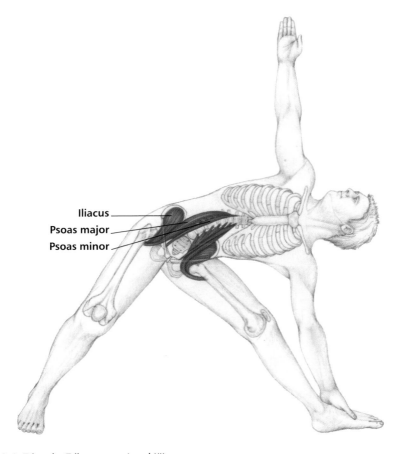

Iliacus
Psoas major
Psoas minor

*Figure 9.4: Triangle, Trikonasana, Level I/II.*

VIII. Half Moon, ***Ardha Chandrasana***, Level II
(*ardha* = half; *chandra* = moon)

A great hip opener and a one-leg support, this pose calls upon the psoas to engage deeply in balancing the body, among other things. The sacral nerve plexus is massaged.

**Technique**: One can get to this pose by starting from Warrior I or II. The arms reach to the floor or a block, and the back leg lifts behind as the front leg straightens. The hips open; the top arm can be placed on the hip, or raised straight up.

**Limitations**: One-leg balances are difficult, but effective. Strength of the bottom leg and flexibility of the top leg are improved with time. Using a wall for support of the back of the body is beneficial for feeling what the pose can achieve. Place the bottom hand on a block support if reaching the floor with a straight bottom leg is difficult.

## Backbends

IX. Bridge Pose, *Setu Bandhasana*, Level I (see illustration on page 42 and 67). (*setu* = dam or bridge; *bandha* = lock)

This pose will open the front of the body and affect both chakras 2 and 3. It is considered a gentle backbend, opening the front hips, abdominals, chest, and heart. The psoas is stretched at the hip.

**Technique**: Lie on the back with the knees bent, feet flat on the floor, hip width apart. The arms can be along the sides of the body as the hips are pushed up off the floor. Once the hips are high enough, the hands can be placed at the hips, or extended under the body with clasped hands. The shoulder blades should remain connected to the floor; this will reduce excessive hyperextension of the spine, and also limit weight on the head and neck. To return, roll down slowly through the spine, exhaling deeply.

**Limitations**: Tight hip flexors (the muscles at the front of the hip joint) will limit the stretch, as well as tight quadriceps on the front thigh that work the knee joint. Easing into the posture will begin to loosen the anterior muscles.

X. Pigeon, *Eka Pada Kapotasana*, Level II
(*eka* = one; *pada* = foot, leg; *kapota* = pigeon, dove)

Another great hip opener, this pose will stretch the psoas to the extreme in the back leg, and help stabilize the spine in an upright position. Affect the sacral chakra by breathing into the lower back and belly, and focusing on the area. The piriformis muscle (mentioned before as a culprit in sciatica when it is tight) will get a nice stretch in the front leg if the posture is forward.

**Technique**: There are a few ways to get into this posture: try starting from table position (all fours). Slide one knee between the hands, placing the foot outside the other hip. Extend the back leg, keeping the hands pressed into the floor for support. Straighten the spine with a "proud chest," with shoulders back and down. Figure 9.5 shows the forward variation.

**Limitations**: Tight hips will inhibit the posture. Try placing a blanket or block under the hip. The core muscles must be engaged when the spine is upright.

Once these postures are completed, the Happy Baby will be a great relaxing pose, opening up the sacrum and lower back.

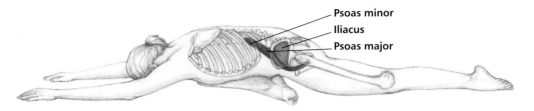

Figure 9.5: Pigeon, Eka Pada Kapotasana, Level II.

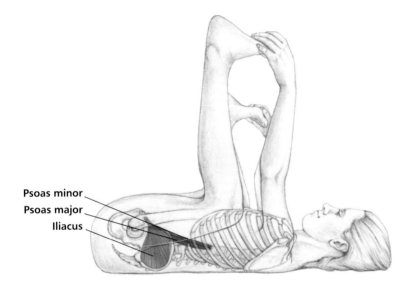

Figure 9.6: Happy Baby, Ananda Balasana, Level I.

The sacral area is best served by honoring relationships and establishing positive emotional and sensual connections. The upper intestines, stomach, liver, gallbladder, kidneys, spleen, pancreas, and adrenal glands are all situated here as well as the psoas and other tissue explained earlier. *Stimulating this sacred place is learning how to flow (like water) and open up to pleasure, without resistance. It is the womb itself, allowing movement and change when healthy.*

## Pointers for Chakra 2

1. Cool down and allow energy to go inward.

2. Receive, accept, and adapt.

3. Eat sweet fruits such as melons, oranges, and coconuts; nuts and honey, as well as spices such as cinnamon, vanilla, and carob, are positive reinforcements.

4. Embrace the feminine qualities of openness, intimacy, and vision.

5. Be creative and let things "circulate."

6. Feel at ease with the body.

7. Learn to let go.

## Bonus Poses

Cat, *Bidalasana/*Cow, *Bitilasana,* Level I

Sometimes called Cat/Dog, this sequence initiates movement from the sacral core, articulating the spine and coordinating movement with breath. Begin on all fours (table position) with a neutral spine. Exhale as the core is lifted against the spine, and round the back by dropping the tailbone and head. Reverse the spinal position by lifting the tailbone and chest on the inhalation. Allow the movement to flow without resistance, like water, beginning at the tailbone.

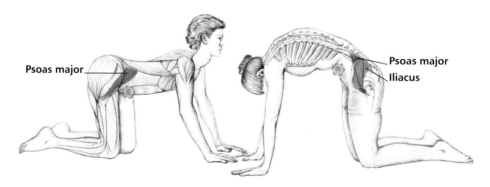

*Figure 9.7: Cat, Bidalasana/Cow, Bitilasana, Level I.*

Crescent, *Anjaneyasana,* Level I: A variety of this posture is shown on page 43. A great psoas lengthener on the back leg side, and groin opener: from a lunge, drop the back knee and rest hands on front thigh, or raise high for more stretch. The core and lumbar spine are stabilizing. For challenge, add lateral flexion (side bending) and/or rotation of the spine or (backbending).

# 10

# The Psoas and
# Chakra 3:
# "Function Meets
# Breath"

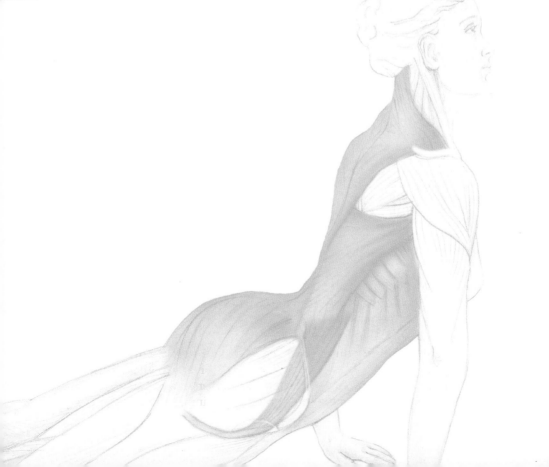

## Yoga Poses and Chakra 3

The third chakra is the solar plexus, an interesting central spot around the naval, full of muscles (psoas, diaphragm), organs (lungs, upper stomach and intestines), and spiritualism. Solar plexus is really not so much an anatomical term; it is more important as an energy and nerve center. It is connected with consciousness of self within the universe, self-knowing and loving. It is where the emotional joins the mental in understanding.

As discussed in Part I, the psoas and diaphragm come together at this junction point. "Function meets breath" would be appropriate here. A very powerful place, this chakra will be stimulated by the following yoga postures, aiding in self-esteem.

## Backbends

I. Cobra Pose, ***Bhujangasana***, Level I
(*bhujanga* = snake; *bhuja* = arm; *anga* = limb)

**Technique**: Lie on the stomach, face down (prone), with hands under the shoulders and elbows in. Extend the legs, pushing the tops of the feet into the floor. Drawing the shoulders back, lift the head and chest using the upper back muscles, not the hands. The hips remain on the floor. Engage the core and breath deeply to massage the psoas.

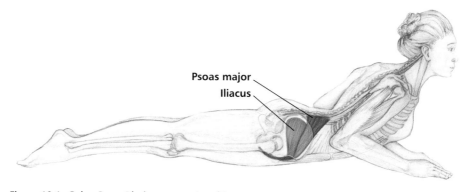

Psoas major
Iliacus

*Figure 10.1: Cobra Pose, Bhujangasana, Level I.*

**Limitations**: Raising the head too far back will compress the cervical vertebrae, so is not advised. Raising the chest too high might result in lower back pain; engage the core to support it.

II. Camel Pose, *Ustrasana*, Level I/II
(*ustra* = camel)

This is a strong front hip opener, stretching the psoas area at the front of the hip.

**Technique**: Begin kneeling, with the legs slightly apart, a straight spine, and hands on hips. Curve the thoracic spine back without pushing the hips forward. Extend the neck, but do not strain it. Lift the rib cage and sternum. The hips should be over the knees. If balanced and the core is engaged, reach the hands toward the heels. One may also curl the toes under on the mat for support.

**Limitations**: Follow the limitations for the Cobra above. If one has trouble with the knees, rest them on a soft support. If this is not possible, do the Cobra as an alternative. Do not arch deeply into the lower spine; squeezing the buttocks and lifting the core will help. One can also use a chair behind to place the hands on.

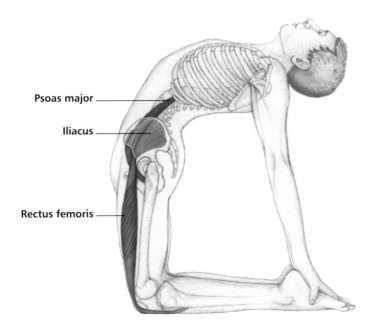

*Figure 10.2: Camel Pose, Ustrasana, Levels I/II.*

III. Upward Facing Dog, *Urdhva Mukha Svanasana*, Level II
(*urdhva* = raised; *mukha* = face; *svana* = dog)

This pose can be done in a simple way, but becomes more advanced when the knees are lifted off the floor. The core is powerfully engaged; the front of the hips and lower psoas are stretched.

**Technique**: Lie face down. Begin as in the Cobra, with the legs spread a bit further apart. Lift the head, chest, and hips off the floor, with the core engaged. If the core is strong, lift the knees also. Foundation points are the dorsal side of the foot (top side) and the hands, with straight elbows. Rotate the shoulders outward to open, dropping the shoulder blades down and in. Extend the neck.

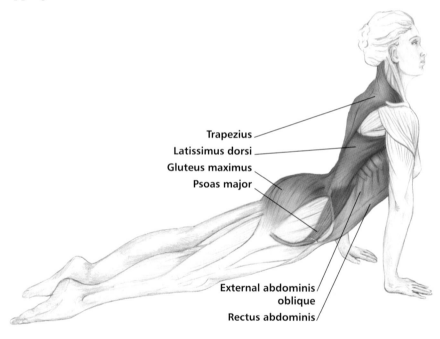

Trapezius
Latissimus dorsi
Gluteus maximus
Psoas major

External abdominis
oblique
Rectus abdominis

*Figure 10.3: Upward Facing Dog, Urdhva Mukha Svanasana, Level II.*

**Limitations**: This pose is difficult because of stress on the arms, cervical spine, and lumbar spine. Look forward, engage the psoas, and keep the knees on the floor to counteract the stress. One can also rest on the elbows, for Sphinx Pose.

IV. Fish Pose, *Matsyasana*, Level II is shown.
(*matsya* = fish)

This pose opens the solar plexus and the heart, as most backbends do. Its effort is concentrated on hyperextension of the middle spine, stretching the diaphragm and abdominals.

**Technique for Level I/II**: Lie on the back (supine) and position the hands under the sacrum and tailbone. Lift the sternum, rest on the forearms, and slowly allow the head to fall back, either resting on the floor or hanging toward or on a support. Draw the shoulder blades toward one another (adduct and retract), which opens the front rib cage. The knees can be bent (Level I), or they can be straightened (Level II) to allow space in the pelvic region. Relax and breathe calmly.

**Technique for Level III**: Lift the arms and/or legs. This can be very difficult for the lower back – remember to listen to the body and be aware of what might be harmful to it.

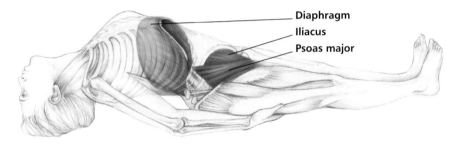

Diaphragm
Iliacus
Psoas major

*Figure 10.4: Fish Pose, Matsyasana, Level II.*

**Limitations**: Opening the heart, rib cage, and throat is hard for many people, but necessary in this age of computers, where a closed chest is the norm. Place a block or blanket under the thoracic spine and head to help relax and stretch the area without strain.

V. Bow Pose, *Dhanurasana,* Level II/III
(*dhanu* = bow)

**Technique**: Lie on the belly, stretched, in prone position. Bend the knees and grab the ankles with both hands, if possible. Bring the head and chest up as well as the thighs. The spine will hyperextend, and the front shoulders will stretch. The lower psoas and rectus abdominis will be fully stretched.

**Limitations**: The front of the shoulder joint is very vulnerable as it is stretched to capacity. Pull the shoulder blades together (adduct and retract) to help reduce strain. The spine can also be taxed in this anterior curve position, so care must be taken not to overdo hyperextension. Separating the knees will lessen strain.

## Inversions

VI. Downward Facing Dog, *Adho Mukha Svanasana,* Level I/II
(*adho* = downward; *mukha* = face; *svana* = dog)

This is one of the most popular, effective, and restful poses in yoga. (Watch a dog perform it naturally when it gets up from resting.) Spine alignment is maintained as the back of the body stretches. This may not sound or feel like rest, but eventually it is. The psoas is released, yet stabilizing, and the diaphragm is open and stretched. Inversions aid blood flow to the brain. The hamstrings and shoulders will be stretched. The naval center supports the lower back when engaged.

**Technique**: Begin in the table position, on hands and knees. Tuck the toes under, engage the naval center, lift the knees, and press the weight back into the legs as the arms and knees straighten and the head drops. Turn the shoulders outward, slide the shoulder blades down the spine, and let the head hang freely. Press the heels toward the floor – but they do not have to touch.

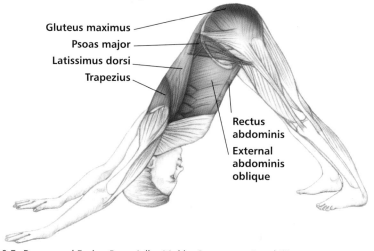

Gluteus maximus
Psoas major
Latissimus dorsi
Trapezius
Rectus abdominis
External abdominis oblique

*Figure 10.5: Downward Facing Dog, Adho Mukha Svanasana, Level I/II.*

**Limitations**: Tight hamstrings and weak shoulders will limit the ease of the pose. Outwardly rotating the shoulders and keeping them away from the ears will help alleviate impingement at the joint. Bent knees will relax the hamstrings. Release tension in the neck by allowing the heavy head to hang freely, as gravity allows, or rest the head on a blanket or block for support. If shoulders are tight, rest on the elbows, for Dolphin Pose.

VII. Sun Salutation, *Surya Namaskar*, Level I
(*surya* = sun; *namaskar* = salute)

This incorporates stretching, strengthening, and relaxation of the psoas, and can bring focus to the third chakra:

1. Begin in Mountain Pose.
2. Inhale to Crescent Stretch: bring the arms overhead and stretch to the sky.
3. Exhale and release to Forward Bend.
4. Inhale, lifting the spine to a flat back position, with the hands on the shins.
5. Exhale to Forward Bend.
6. Inhale and take one leg back to a lunge position.
7. Exhale and take the other leg back to Plank (push-up position) and lower the body to the floor.
8. Inhale to Cobra.
9. Exhale to Child's Pose. Rest for three full breaths.
10. Inhale to table position.
11. Exhale to Down Dog. Rest for three long, full breaths: ocean (*ujjayi*) breath.
12. Inhale, walking or jumping the feet to between the hands.
13. Exhale to Forward Bend , inhale and do number 4, then exhale back to Forward Bend.
14. Inhale to roll up the spine, raising the arms to the sky.
15. Exhale to Mountain Pose (hands in *Namaste*, prayer position, centering, sealing the practice).

All movements in the Sun Salutation will ground the spirit to the earth (chakra 1), flow the body with the breath (chakras 2 and 3), and release tension as the body warms and opens up.

*Keep in mind, the best way to learn* asanas (postures) is by taking a *yoga class with a certified instructor from a legitimate yoga school.*

Any abdominal strength exercise will also stimulate the third chakra. Strengthening the core creates vitality and self-esteem. Be careful not to perfect this area too much though, as it will lead to feelings of power over others, instead of empowerment. Balance is the key, without overworking.

Eating grains, dairy or soy, and herbs such as mint will nourish this area. Digestive troubles, eating and metabolism disorders, and even arthritis are issues associated with this chakra. Creating a healthy, balanced solar plexus helps assert one's will and assume responsibility without fear.

## Pointers for Chakra 3

1.  Breathe deeply.

2.  Do some nice, full, belly-laughing.

3.  Perform selfless services; volunteer.

4.  Pay attention to your energy levels.

5.  Nourish yourself.

6.  Take risks.

7. Empower the core.

## The True Bonus Pose: *Savasana*

Corpse Pose, *Savasana*, Level 1
(*sava* = corpse)

This is the easiest *asana* to perform but the hardest to master – the challenge is to let go. Tension must be completely released from the body and mind while lying on the back, legs slightly apart, arms out from sides with palms turned up; eyes are closed. Surrender is a term that has the connotation of something negative in today's society, as in "giving up." In yoga it is highly respected as one submits and opens to the rhythms of the cosmos. This is the state of a true yogi.

From a friend and colleague, Irum Naqvi*:

*Surrender is a most beautiful word. It is powerful and nurturing, healing us as it provides both strength and compassion.*

*As we understand the essence and meaning of the word* surrender *through our hearts, we begin to transform. As we transform internally the external world changes. "As within, so without."*

*How to surrender is many faceted. The word itself has two parts. First we begin to release what is held by the mind, body, and spirit. The release can be facilitated through focus and breath awareness. Along with this focus, the breath is brought to the forefront, using the breath as the guide in scanning the physical sensations, mental thoughts, and emotional feelings.*

*With the release, an acceptance of "what is" happening is important. When we release and accept and embrace life in any moment, we are surrendering. It leaves us open to the moment, to being completely present. With continuous practice of surrendering we build the ability to heal. As we heal, the space that opens up is filled with joy.*

*Surrender, heal, and be in joy.*

*Irum B. Naqvi has been practicing yoga for more than 20 years; she is a yoga alliance certified teacher and a Reiki practitioner. Irum has taught yoga in Austria, the UK, Canada, and Costa Rica. Currently she resides at the beautiful Rancho Margot in Costa Rica, teaching yoga and sponsoring yoga teacher trainings. Rancho Margot is an ecotourism ranch project where the author and Irum plan to sponsor yoga retreats in the future. http://www.ranchomargot.org*

There is a "plethora of slightly inaccurate information out there" (quoted from a master Kundalini teacher) as the fields of exercise, yoga, and meditation constantly evolve and integrate. Hopefully this text has explained it in a most sincere and simple way, without attention to any particular school of thought.

**Yoga postures connect the body to the mind.**

**Breathing connects the mind and body to the unconscious.**

**Meditation connects the person to the universe.**

**The psoas major connects the upper body to the lower body, linking breath to movement, feelings, energy, and healing.**

*PART 3*

*Chapter 10 – The Psoas and Chakra 3: "Function Meets Breath"*

# Appendix: The Hip Flexion Society

Ask yourself the following questions:

1. Do you use a computer?
2. Do you drive or ride in a car?
3. Do you watch TV?
4. Do you read?
5. Do you sit at a table to eat?
6. Do you play cards or video games?
7. Do you go to the movies?
8. Are you a student?
9. Do you write?
10. Do you fly a lot?

If you answered yes to some of the above questions, you are a member of the "hip flexion society" – a civilization that is becoming more sedentary than during any other time period in history, because it spends a lot of time sitting in chairs. The next thing to determine is how many hours a day you sit. It may startle you.

Sitting is a relaxed hip flexion position: relaxed, because the hip flexor muscles are not working against resistance (contracting) – they are merely in a flexed state, with the full weight of the torso above seated into the pelvic floor, and the lower extremities inactive. It is a position which, if held too long, will inhibit circulation, muscle conditioning, and even nerve response. It can be a direct cause of lower back, psoas, and sciatic issues; the hip flexors begin to shorten and weaken, and over time create a myriad of problems.

## Case Study

I recently did a month-long study with 12 adult volunteers – 3 men and 9 women, myself included. The study was based on the hip flexors, and was meant to include awareness of the psoas muscle as part of the iliopsoas system, the deepest hip flexor muscle group. The participants were to complete, 3–4 times weekly for 4 weeks, a 10-minute stretch and strength routine which targeted the hip flexors.*

Measurements were taken before and after to compare the strength, endurance, and flexibility of the hip flexor region. Although results were positive (albeit inconclusive as to the effect of the routine), the biggest surprise to all was the amount of sitting they did daily. I asked each of them to document how many hours they sat on the days they did the exercise, as well as any other exercise. The numbers were shocking: those that completed the study recorded a minimum of 5 hours a day sitting, and a maximum of 11, depending on the day. These were working adults who live in the northeastern part of the United States, where commuting and computer work are almost obligatory.

* To view the 10-minute hip flexor exercise routine, e-mail the author at: movetolive.joannjones@gmail.com

The hip flexor case study led me to wonder about young students in school. They are typically a high-energy group with physical activity (mostly sports) available to them, so how much time do they spend sitting? Once again, results are astounding. For children in school, the sitting time varies from 5 to 8 hours; they usually go home by car or bus and then sit at the computer, hopefully do homework, and perhaps watch TV, all of which involve sitting. While at school, they are sometimes given a reprieve by getting up to change classrooms, which usually has a time limit of 3 minutes before they have to sit again. On top of all this, the normal recess or physical education pilot class is in jeopardy of being eliminated from school programs.

There are some common-sense approaches for dealing with the increasingly devastating problem of too much hip flexion, for both children and adults:

1. If sitting, get up once every hour and stretch in all directions.
2. Design a computer space where you can stand while working. Make sure the monitor is at eye level.
3. Play video games that involve body movement.
4. Take a yoga class.** This involves hip flexion, but it is counteracted by stretching.
5. Go for a walk.
6. Sit less and move more.

Another remedy is to stretch the body out while reading or gazing at the TV. If lying on the back, care should be taken to make sure the spine is neutral. Put a pillow under the knees, and prop the head up a bit by supporting the neck with a pillow or towel. When lying on the stomach, the hip flexors will stretch, which is good; however, the lower back will compress, so this position should not be held for long, and the core should engage to protect the spine. Moreover, the neck is in a compromised position of hyperextension while you are trying to look up at something, so this position is not ideal.

Likewise, not the best solutions for too much sitting are some very valid conditioning programs where you are moving, but there is too much hip flexion. Be careful in aerobics, Pilates, and kickboxing, and on many workout machines. Make sure that not only is there the counteraction of hip extension, but there is also movement that happens in all three planes: sagittal (front and back), frontal (side to side), and horizontal (rotation).

** In the large city of Newark, NJ, there is a public school pilot program that includes yoga in every student's experience, to aid in movement as well as outlook. (Imagine how this might reduce violence in inner-city neighborhoods someday.) www.newarkyogamovement.org